Technology and Nutritional View of Yoghurt

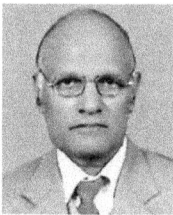

The Author

Dr. Jai Singh presently working as Professor and Former Head, Department of Animal Husbandry and Dairying, Institute of Agricultural Sciences, Banaras Hindu University, Varanasi. Dr. Singh has more than 27 years of teaching and research experiences of undergraduate and postgraduate levels. He has published several research papers in International Journals of repute and authored five books. Besides this, he has guided more than 30 M.Sc. and Ph.D. students. Dr. Singh has participated/ delivered lectures at various National and International Conferences and Symposium. Dr. Singh is recipient of several awards and fellowships by various scientific societies for his outstanding contributions in the field of Animal Husbandry and Dairying.

Technology and Nutritional View of Yoghurt

Dr. Jai Singh

Professor
Former Head
Department of Animal Husbandry and Dairying
Institute of Agricultural Sciences
Banaras Hindu University
Varanasi - 221005

2015

Daya Publishing House®
A Division of
Astral International (P) Ltd
New Delhi 110 002

Cataloging in Publication Data—DK
Courtesy: D.K. Agencies (P) Ltd. <docinfo@dkagencies.com>

Singh, Jai *(Professor of animal husbandry and dairying),* **author.**
  Technology and nutritional view of yoghurt / Dr. Jai Singh.
    pages   cm
  Includes bibliographical references (pages   ).

  ISBN 978-93-5130-747-1 (International Edition)

    1. Yogurt. 2. Yogurt—Health aspects. 3. Dairy processing—
  Technological innovations. 4. Dairying.   I. Title.

DDC 637.146   23

Published by   : **Daya Publishing House**®
                          A Division of
                          Astral International Pvt. Ltd.
                          – ISO 9001:2008 Certified Company –
                          4760-61/23, Ansari Road, Darya Ganj
                          New Delhi-110 002
                          Ph. 011-43549197, 23278134
                          E-mail: info@astralint.com
                          Website: www.astralint.com

Laser Typesetting   : **Classic Computer Services**, Delhi - 110 035

Printed at   : **Thomson Press India Limited**

PRINTED IN INDIA

PREFACE

India is predominately an agricultural country and the dairying recognized as an instrument for social and economic development because milk is the largest crop after rice in India agriculture. At present dairy industry has achieved tremendous progress in the country with surplus stock of milk in some dairy of the states of India. The quantum of research information is so vast on the subject of dairy technology that it would be in insurmountable task to comprehand, compile and present it in a single book.

The text book written on yoghurt by eminant teachers and scientists are in limited dimention. No single text book caters the needs of under graduates, graduates students and research workers of dairy science and dairy technology in the country by providing all the needful information comprehesively on "Technology and Nutritional value of yoghurt" at a single source.

The basic approach in preparing the contents of the book is in tune with the current thinking on the subject and furthering its pursuit by strenthening the knowledge and understanding based on the rapidly advancing newer concept and discoveries. Keeping the ultimate size the completion in mind, it was necessary to condense the voluminous literature without sacrificing the originality of concept, old and new.

Special appreciation is due to author's family members and friends for their cooperation and patience during completion of the book.

Jai Singh

CONTENTS

Objectives, heat transfer for fluid milk, pasteurization, thermization, sterilization. UHT processing. use of microwave technology. BIS standard for UHT milk homogenization principles and effect of heat on physico-chemical properties of milk.

Additives and lactic acid bacteriafood colouring agents. natural flavouring agents, agents stabilizers. perspective and stages of addition of additives. Species of lactic acid bacteria characteristics and importance of lactic acid bacteria.

Internal challenges. Food hazards, hazard analysis and critical control points (HACCP), benefits of HACCP, Total quality management, meeting the challenges of quality, BIS standards for dahi and yoghurt.

Purpose, Functions, criteria to judge the packaging, forms of packaging materials, reasons for use of plastics for packaging. Modified atmosphere packaging, advantages and disadvantages of MAP, aseptic package.

Effect of milk on physico-chemical quality of yoghurt, (2) Effect of fat and SNF on physico-chemical quality of yoghurt, (3) Effect of starter culture and incubation temperature on physico-chemical quality of yoghurt and (4) Effect of feeding yoghurt on growth rate, feed efficiency and blood profile in rats.

1 Introduction

The momentous task of restructuring dairy industry in India on modern line began about 42 years ago. In the absence of industrial experience with techno-economic and climatic conditioning the early growth is mainly involved transporting of western technologies to the Indian situation. Thus, refrigeration was introduced for collection and transportation of raw milk from rural areas to the dairy plants, pasteurization was adopted for processing market milk for urban consumption, and a number of western products were introduced to balance regional and seasonal fluctuation of milk production. Efforts made so far has resulted in developing capabilities for processing about 12-15% of the total milk produced in India through about 580 dairy factories in the co-operative, public and private sector.

In past three decades, India has achieved a tremendous growth in the field of dairy. In terms of milk production, as also in annual growth in production, the country's performance has been apparent. It is very well established fact that dairying has benefited the poor maximum as compared to any other sector of the Indian economy. On an average about 22.5% of income of rural households, is contributed by milk, during the past 50 years, although the contribution of agriculture sector to the GDP of the country, as whole, has come down drastically, the live stock sector has been able to maintain its contribution to the GDP more or less at the same level.

Inspite of the such phenomenal growth, we are far below the world average in terms of productivity, while India has 2.0% of the geographical area of the world, it supports about 18% of world's cattle and buffalo population but contributes only about 14% of the milk output. Thus, even to be considered at par with world's average productivity level. we should have to produced over 125 million tonnes of milk as compared to about 112 million tonnes which we are producing now.

The dairy industry has helped the national economy by making us position as the highest milk producing country in the world. Today, milk is the leading agricultural produce contributing 7.0 per cent of the India's GDP. The unique feature of the system is that 70 millions of rural farmers are engaged in milk production as against large specialized dairy farmers in the western country. With the initiation of Operation Flood Programme, launched in 1970, under the aegies of National Dairy Development Board (NDDB), we have come a long way and has been able to raise the per capita availability of milk to 290 gm as against the minimum requirement of 280 gm as recommended by ICMR, New Delhi. This is really achievement considering spiraling rise in human population.

India which once used to import milk, rank first in the world total milk production. Milk production in India has been increasing steadily during the last five years at the rate of 4.0-4.5 per cent annually. The total milk production in India has grown at an average annual compound rate of 5.15 per cent during 1980-81 to 1990-91 and at 4.06 per cent during 1990-91 to 1998-99. The annual per capita availability of milk in the country has grown at the rate of 3.02 per cent annually during 1980-81 to 1990-91 (Sazena, 2000).

About 45 per cent of milk produced is consumed as liquid milk and the remainder converted into a wide range of dairy products (28% ghee, 7% dahi, 6.5% khoa, 6.5% butter, 2.6% milk powder, 2.0% chhana, cheese and panner, 0.50% cream, 0.2% ice cream and 1.7% others).

The process of the souring or fermentation of milk is one of the oldest method to preserve milk. Basically all fermented milk products are made through addition of appropriate starter culture to milk followed by development of acidity to the desired level. In the process of fermentation lactic acid plays an essential role in the milk. It exerts an antagonistic impact on harmful microbes let alone it action to transforming the substrate into a new products both at the domestic and industrial levels. Different micro-organisms and their mixed cultures are used globally to carry out the fermentation process. This results in a wide range of well known and well documented fermented milk products *viz.*, the name of products are also varied with the change manufacturing process and addition of cereals during manufacturing of products *viz.* kumiss, kefir, dahi, acidophilus milk, bulgarican milk, yoghurt etc. (Table - 1). The name of product are also varied with the change of manufacturing process and addition of cereals during manufacturing of products (fig.1). Among the various microbiol cultures microbial cultures used for dairy products, yoghurt has gained paramount importance. The word yoghurt derived from the Turkish word, 'Jughurt'. Yoghurt is a traditional food and beverage among Balkans of the middle-east. However, its popularity has now spread to Europe and to many other parts of the world and its consumption has increased significantly during the past three decades.

Out of all dairy products, the fermented milk and milk products, especially yoghurt seems to have a very important role and place in the diet of human being a highly refreshing, nutritious and healthful food drink. Yoghurt has been developed over thousand of years around the mediterranean basin, the middle-east and India. The product is known as laban or laben (in Lebanon and most neighbouring countries), laben (in Morocco), dahi (in India), and zabadi (in Ezypt). It was originated in eastern Europe, even today, the per capita consumption of yoghurt is more than 10 times greater in Europe than in the United States. Despite the different spelling used (hoghurt, yoghurt, yahourt, yaourt, Laben, Madzoon and Naya etc). Yoghurt is a wide spread product. Commercial production of yoghurt increased rapidly in 20th century and attempts to popularize yoghurt in the United States and Canada, were successful in 1940s.

Table1 : Traditional Fermented milks*

S.No.	Name of the Country	Name of products
1.	Arab countries	Labmehand and lebmeh
2.	Armeria	Katyk, matsun, matzoon, madzoon, tass and than
3.	Bulgaria	Yoghurt
4.	Greece	Tiaoruti
5.	Hungary	Tarho
6.	India	Dahi
7.	Indonesia	Dadih
8.	Fran	Dough, mask, masg and mast
9.	Iraqe	Laban, Leben, naja, rob and robia
10.	Lebanon	Jubjub, labnesh and lebneh
11.	Nepal	Dahi
12.	Russia	Koumiss and kefir
13.	Saudi Arabia	Laban rayeb
14.	Sudan	Naja, rob, robia, zabade and zabadi
15.	Turkey	Ayran, Kurute, torba, tulum and yoghurt

Kosikowsky (1966) and Goldin (1980)

In the production of yoghurt generally mixed culture of specific microbial species are used. The use of specific microbial species in the manufacture of this product improves its quality, provides uniformity and helps to standardized this product on specific lines in addition to render them clean and safe for human consumption. Thus, it deals with the significance of various microbes associated with the dairy products in human nutrition.

The major beneficial changes associated with yoghurt includes alteration in protein, metabolic products formed from lactose and hydrolytic changes occurring in the milk fat. The final product is rendered more digestible. As calcium is free from caseinogen in the milk, it combines with lactic acid to form calcium lactate which is easily assimilable. The yoghurt contains more thiamine and riboflavin tham fresh milk.

Yoghurt (Bulgaria, Turkey), tiaourti (Greece) gioddu (Sardinia), mesolada (Sicily), leben (Iraq) rawbah (Iraq), Sudan, Saudi Arabia), laban (Syria, Lebanon, Jordan), lebben (Israel), laban rayeh (Saudi Arabia), zabady (Egypt, Sudan), mast Iran

Dilute — Ayran (Turkey), dough (Iran)

Add — Dry — Kushuk (Iraq), kichk (Lebanon), trahana (Greece) cereals

Remove water — Torba (Turkey), tulum yoghurt (Turkey), labaneh (Jordan), labeniah (Israel), labneh (Syria, Saudi Arabia), labaneh anbaris (Lebanon), laban zeer (Egypt)

Dry — Kurut (Turkey), jubjub (Lebanon), duberki (israel), jamid (Jordan)

Add — Dry — Kishk (Egypt) cereals

Heat — Winter yoghurt (Turkey) concentration

Stir — Tere ya (Turkey)

Ayan (Turkey), laban khad (Egypt), butter dough (Iran), doug (Afghanistan)

Remove water — Lebenen bezt (Syria), Chaka (Afghanistan)

Dry — Kachk (Iran), krut (Afghanistan)

Heat to remove water — Chokerek (Turkey), kasshk (Iran)

Dry — Karabesch (Iran), aoules (Algeria)

Add — Dry — Kishk (Egypt) cereals

Milk

Culture

Fermented milk

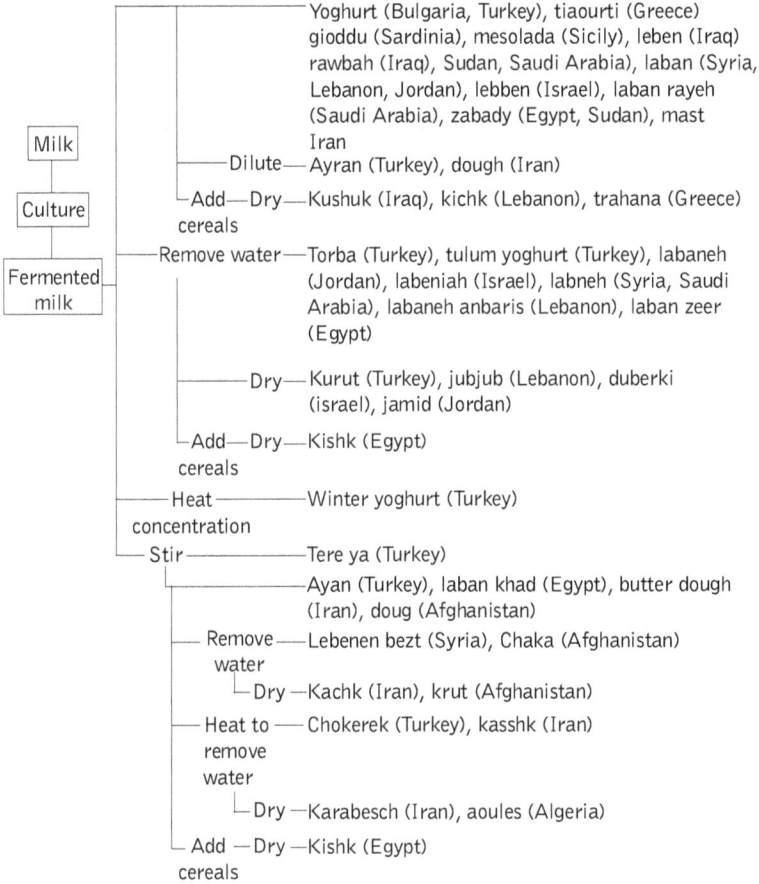

Fig. 1: Fermented milk products in and around the Middle and Near East

Growth of *Streptococcus thermophilus* is stimulated by amino acids, principally valine, liberated by *Lactobacillus bulgaricus*. *S. thermophilus* liberates the formic acid which stimulates the growth of *L.bulgaricus*.

Yoghurt has sharp characteristic acid flavour and smooth texture which are important quality aspect of the product. It possess a high viscosity producing a smooth pleasant sensation on the palate.

The quality of final product always depends on the quality of raw materials (mostly milk and culture). Since in yoghurt, milk and culture are the two main raw materials, so the quality of these two materials should be good enough to produce a quality product. The quality of yoghurt also depends on the treatment of the milk which include optimum level of fat and SNF, techniques of homogenization and extent of heat treatment. Another important aspect of yoghurt manufacture is the unique bacterial fermentation by right type and amount of bacterial cultures.

The physical properties of coagulum are primarily dependent on casein and non-casein ratio. High heat treatment of the milk used in manufacturing the yoghurt, is essential to denature whey protein, thus increasing the capacity of protein to bind water and liberate amino acids that promote growth of *L.bulgaricus* enzymatically, hydrolyses protein providing amino acids, especially valine, that making the growth of *S. thermophilus*. *S. thermophilus* uses oxygen, thus making the oxygen tension more favourable for *L.bulgaricus*. It is very clear that *S. thermophilus* liberates the formic acid which stimulate the growth of *L. bulgaricus.*

Cow milk is generally used for manufacture of yoghurt. It may also be manufactured from goat, sheep and baffalo milk. Yoghurt is available in many types and varieties, but the board categories are natural and plain yoghurt (stirred and set yoghurt), flavoured yoghurt (both stirred and set), sweetened flavoured yoghurt, fruit flavoured yoghurt (both stirred and set), sweetened flavoured yoghurt, fruit flavoured yoghurt. For high quality, yoghurt should have fresh appearance, custured like with a smooth texture, light sourish taste with natural yoghurt flavour. Normally 0.8 to 1.0 per cent lactic acid desired in the product.

Fermented milk product play an important role in the prevention of gastrointestinal disorders like diarrhoea etc., suppresses tumour growth, deceases the chances of cancer besides lowering the blood cholesterol levels. Yoghurt has the important value for those who possess the problem of lactose intolerance. This often results due to reduced lactase activity in the intestinal tract. In yoghurt lactose level is considerably reduced. Yoghurt contains substantial amount of lactase bounded to the cell of microbes which might also be contribute to intestinal hydrolysis of lactose after consumption of yoghurt.

The appropriate scientific information about different levels of bacterial culture, compositional quality of milk, levels of temperature etc., in the preparation of yoghurt and their nutritional impact are not available in our country. Looking the above facts the present book is partly based on the research conducted (kumar, 2002)on the following points:

1. The effect of sources of milk, different levels of fat, SNF, incubation temperature and bacterial cultures on flavour, body and texture, acidity score and colour & appearance of the product.

2. The effect of different factors viz. sources of milk, fat, SNF incubation temperature and bacterial cultures on the chemical quality of the product viz., fat, protein, lactose, ash, acidity and pH.

3. To select the best qualtily yoghurt evolved out of the different treatment combinations tried.

4. Effect of yoghurt on feed efficiency and growth rate in rats.

5. The impact of yoghurt on serum cholesterol, serum triglyceride, serum phospholipid and serum glucose in the rat.

2 Heat Treatment

Objectives

1. To provide safety : After killing pathogenes like mycobacterium tuberculosis, Salmonella species, Staphylococcus aureus, Coxiella burnetii etc. provide safety to the consumers.

2. To Inhance keeping quality : After killing the spoilage causing organisms and their sporces, and inactivation of enzymes present in the milk (native and microbial origine).

3. To establishing desirable properties of specific products : Bactofugated milk is not of good character if it is not free or incativated from bacterial inhibitor (like immunoglobulines and the lactoperoxidase - $CNS-H_2O_2$). This helps in inhance the growth of starter culture bacterial. Inactivation process of these bacterial inhibitor are performed by heat treatment.

4. For preparing desired dairy products : The dairy products like chhana, paneer, cheese, desiccated milk, dried milk etc. can be prepared.

5. To minimise storage space : Dried, condensed or semidried milk products require less space which are easy in transportation than fluid milk.

Heat transfer for fluid Products :

Heat transfer is net transfer of energy from one place to other place due to transfer difference across the boundry. Heat is positive in a situation when the surroundings are at a higher temperature than the system. Heat transfer take place when convention of energy due to temperature difference is present and the system boundry is at solid-fluid interface. To satisfy the convention of energy due to transfer difference the following ceriteria should be fulfilled :

1. Fluid carrier in which conduction accurs is necessary.
2. Fluid should be in contact with solid carrier in which conduction is occuring.
3. Relative motion should be present between the fluid and the solid surface.
4. Transfer difference should exist in the fluid. Convention heat transfer (Qn) is given as :

Convertion, A = area perpendicular to the transfer,

$$Q_n = he\ A\ (T_E - T_S)\ \text{where he = coefficient of}$$

TE = temperature of the surroundings (wall), and

Ts = temperature of the system fluid

An industrial process, heating applications are of the three types:

1. High temperature (above 590^0C)
2. Medium temperature (290 - 590^0C)
3. Low temperature (below 290^0C)

PASTEURIZATION

This type of heat treatment is based on the temperature and time relationship on thermal death time with heat resistant micro-ogranisms (Corelliae burnettii, most heat-resistance pathogen found in milk). On the basis of the relation of temperature and time generally two types of pasteurization process are in practice:

1. Low temperature short time (LTST) - This method is followed for pasteurization of milk in batches.
2. High temperature short time (HTST) - This is an important method for contineous processing of milk. The time and temperature for pasteurization of milk in indirect heat exchangers are given in Table. 1.

Table 1. Time and tempeature relationship for HTST

Temperature		Time
°C	°F	
62.8	145	30 minutes
71.7	161	15 second
88.3	191	1 second
90.0	194	0.5 second
93.9	201	0.1 second
95.6	204	0.05 second
100.0	212	0.01 second

In the pasteurization process all the pathogenes are killed but it is not necessary to kill all the microorganisms present in the fluids. Phosphatase enzyme is completely destroyed at above temperature and time of heating. Presence of phosphatase enzyme is an indication of incomplete pasteurization process of milk.

Thermization

It is a process of heat treatment in which raw milk is heated at 62 to 65°C for 10 to 20 second and cooled to 5°C. This milk can be stored for 3 days without the multiplication of psychrotropic bacteria.

Sterilization

Sterilization process indicates complete destruction of micro-organisms is the milk and milk products through heating process. According to PFA rule, sterilization of milk in our country means heating milk continuosly to temperature of 115°C for 15 minutes or 145°C for 3 second or equivalent temperature time combination to ensure preservation at room temperature for a period of not less than 15 days from the date of manufacture. Additionally the sterilized milk shows absence of albumin by negative terbidity test and it must be sold only in sterilized container. The time necessary to kill all the organisms under specific condition at a specific temperature called *thermal death time* (TDT). The time required for one log cycle reduction of micro-organisms is called *decline_reduction value* (D value). Temperature required for one log change in D value is knows as Z value.

Ultra-high-temperature (UHT) process

The ultra-high-temperature process has been developed during the past 40 years. This is a sterilization process by which treated milk can be stored for longer duration at room temperature. In this process milk is heated to 135^0C-149^0C (275-300^0F) for 2 to 8 seconds.

The heat treatment in UHT is given by two methods :

(i) Direct heating by steam infusion or injection, (ii) Indirect heating where heat is transformed across a heat exchange surface. In former method, steam water is diluted in the milk, so volume of original milk is enhanced. To over come this problem an arrangement for evaporative cooling in vacuum is made. Before giving high temperature milk is heated. This heating process is completed under pressure. The stages of heating are as follows :

5^0C - 55^0C - 130^0C - 140^0C - 75^0C - 25^0C

The above heated milk is packed as such in tetrapack without cooling. The pack contains the following 5 layers:

(i)   Polyethylene
(ii) Paper board
(iii) Polyethylene
(iv) Almunium foil
(v)   Polyethylene

Uses of Microwave technique in dairy processing

1. Dairy products can effectively be sterilized in a suitable form.

2. The self life of the packed product is enhanced under ambient condition.

3. It facilitates uniform and rapid heating of milk and milk products.

4.   It reduces the heat damage to the products.

5.   It attains very high temperature in short time.

BIS standard for UHT milk

1.   Spore/ml of milk - less than 5

2.   Albumin content - negative

3.   Variation in the pH - not more than 0.3 units

4.   Variation in the titrable acidity during 7 days incubation at 550C - not more than 0.02%

Homogenization of milk

In this process fat globules of milk are broken down into smaller size. The diamer of fat globules generally ranges between 2 and 5 μm which is < 1 μm.

Principle of homogenization

The density of fat in milk is lower than other constituents of milk which lead to natural separation of fat. Fat globules in solid state are not broken up. Butter-fat in milk should be in liquid state. The normal melting point of butter fat is 33 °C (91.4°F). The homogenization is more effective at 41 to 71°C (105.8 to 159.8°F) at the speed of 100-400 meters/second. Homogenization takes place at specific pressure (more than 68.9 Mpa) under two to three cylinders (at present 7 or more cylinder models are available). In simple homogenizer the pressure is maintained at 10-25 Mega paskal at 60-70°C with the speed of 100-200 meter/second. The shearing action created in the milk between the homogenizing valve and its sheat reduced the size of fat globules. The size of globules become more uniform as the number of plungers are increased.

Yoghurt and curd (dahi) prepared form homogenized milk are more safer and brighter than products obtained from unhomogenized milk. These products prepared from homogenized milk require less time as compared to other methods.

Effect of heat on the physical and chemical properties of milk

1. Gas from the milk is removed. The extent of removal of gas depends on the type of equipments, time and extent of heating.

2. Enzymes are inactivated.

3. Some vitamins are reduced and lost.

4. Almost all the serum proteins of milk are denatured and turned into soluble form.

5. Sulfhydryl groups of milk proteins are free. It may cause a drop of the redox potential/oxidation-reduction potential.

6. Loss of available lysine due to Maillard reactions (between lactose and protein)

7. Some of the amino acid reduces are changed on intensive heat treatments. They may react with each other and form insoluble components. Some of examples are as follows:

    Glutamine $\rightarrow$ glutamic acid

    Asparagine $\rightarrow$ aspartic acid

    Aspartic acid + Lysine $\rightarrow$ isopeptide

8. Casein micells (αs, $\alpha s2$, β, Y and K casein) accumulated. It may lead to coagulation.

9. Lactose isomarises, part of which may lead to production of organic acid (formic acid).

10. Phoshporic esters of casein are hydrolized and the amount of organic phosphate increases. This may lead to split phospholipids and dissolve ester in the milk.

11. The amount of Ca^{++} decreases and the colloidal phosphate increases upto certain levels at which these changes are reversible but it may slow manner.

12. The titrable acidity of milk enhances and the pH decreases because of increase in organic acid, colloidal phosphate and cleaves of peptide chains and production of soluble peptides etc.

13. The fatty materials are transformed into methyl ketones and lactones.

14. Fat globule membrane are also affected.

Some markable effect of heat on milk

1. **Colour** - Colour of milk may be brown due to Maillard reation.

2. **Appearance** - (a) Creaming appearance of milk may be reduced mainly due to serum protein denaturation.

    (b) Viscosity of milk may increase due to accumulation of casein micelles.

    (c) Rennetability is reduced.

    (d) Heat coagulation and tendency of age thickning decreases.

    (e) Slow heating of milk increases skin formation on the top.

3. **Flavour** - Off-flavour may be developed due to Maillard reaction, formation of free sulphydril groups, accumulation of casein micells and some other reactions of protein.

4. **Survival of bacteria** - Bacterial inhibitors like immunoglobulines and lactoperoxidase - H_2O_2 - CNS become ineffective as a result of which congenial atmosphere may help to survive and grow faster for some of the bacteria in the milk.

5. **Nutritive value** - Due to loss of some important vitamins, Maillard reactions and denaturation of proteins the nutritive value of milk decreased. The biological value of milk proteins decreases significantly as intensity of heating incrases.

3 Yoghurt-Additives and Lactic Acid Bacteria

Yoghurt is a fermented milk product abtained by fermenting milk with the use of lactic acid bacteria or yeast. Yoghurt may be prepared from cow, buffalo, goat, ewe or their mixed milk with or without addition of powdered milk, skin milk or other additives after its fermentation with lactic acid fermentation, using bacteria like *Streptococcus salivarius* ssp. *thermophilus* (*S. thermophilus*) and Lactobacillus delbrvechii ssp. bulgraricus (*L.bulgaricus*). These two bacteria are required for product characteristies espicially flavour. There are some other specific bacteria from which yoghurt may be prepare but the characteristies of the product are singificantly changed (Vedamuthu, 1991). These Optional/additional bacteria are the following:

Lactobacillus acidophilus

L. casei

L. helveticus

L. jugurti

L.lactis

Bifidobacterium bifidum

B. infantis

B. longum

To sweeten the yoghurt 4% sucrose is added in milk without any adverse effect on acid production during its preparation (Vedamuthu 1991). On the basis of International Standard the following additives may be permitted to be incorporated in the milk during Yoghurt preparation :-

(i) Food colouring agents

Acid brilliant green BS, azorubin, Betanin (250), beetroot red, black PN, brilliant black PN (12), C blue No.1, carminic acid (20), carmoisine, cochimeal red A (48), caramel colour 3 (150), Chocolate brown FB (30), chocolate red 2G (30), erythrosine BS (27), ponceau 4R, sunset yellow FCF, Orange yellow 5(12), tartrazine (18) etc.

(ii) Natural flavouring agents

Fruits, fruits juice, chocolate, cocoa, nuts, spices, coffee, honey and other harmless flavours.

(iii) Stabilizers

Agar-Agar, ammonium alginale, arobic gum, bean gum, calcium alginates, carraggeenan, Sodium carboxymethylcellulose (cellulose gum), furcellaran, guar gum, gelatins, Karaya gum, pectins, prohylene glycol alginate, potassium alginate, starehes, sodium alginate, tragacanth gum, xanthan gum.

(iv) Preservatives

Calcium, sodium and potassium sorbates, SO_2, sorbic acid, benzoic acid at buels in the final products resulting from those permitted in the individual codex standards for fruit based products, or upto 50 mg/kg (alone or in combination).

Stages of addition of additives

In soft or stirred yoghurt generally starter is added without stabilizers and colours. It does not have jelly like jel texture, but is highly viscous semi-fluid. In set yoghurt stabilizers an used to strenthen the gel and prevent water separation (wheying off) generally, gelating or agar alone or mixed together are used (Fig. 2). The colouring agents are now being used as per desince of the consumers in both types of yoghurt at the stage mentioned in Fig. 3.1 & 3.2.

Milk (Clean and safe)
↓
Standardization
↓
Pre-heating (55 - 60°C)
↓
Mixing
↓
Homogenization (150kg-200kg/cm²)
↓
Posteurization (HTST or UHT or batch)
↓
Cooling (42 - 48°C)

Starter ────────►|
Flavour ────────►|
if desire   ↓

Mixing
↓
Fill into containers
↓
Fermentation (43-48°C, 3-5hrs)
↓
Cooling
↓
Product
↓ ◄────── **(may be filled in small**
Storage   **containers if so, require**
                     cooling for resetting)

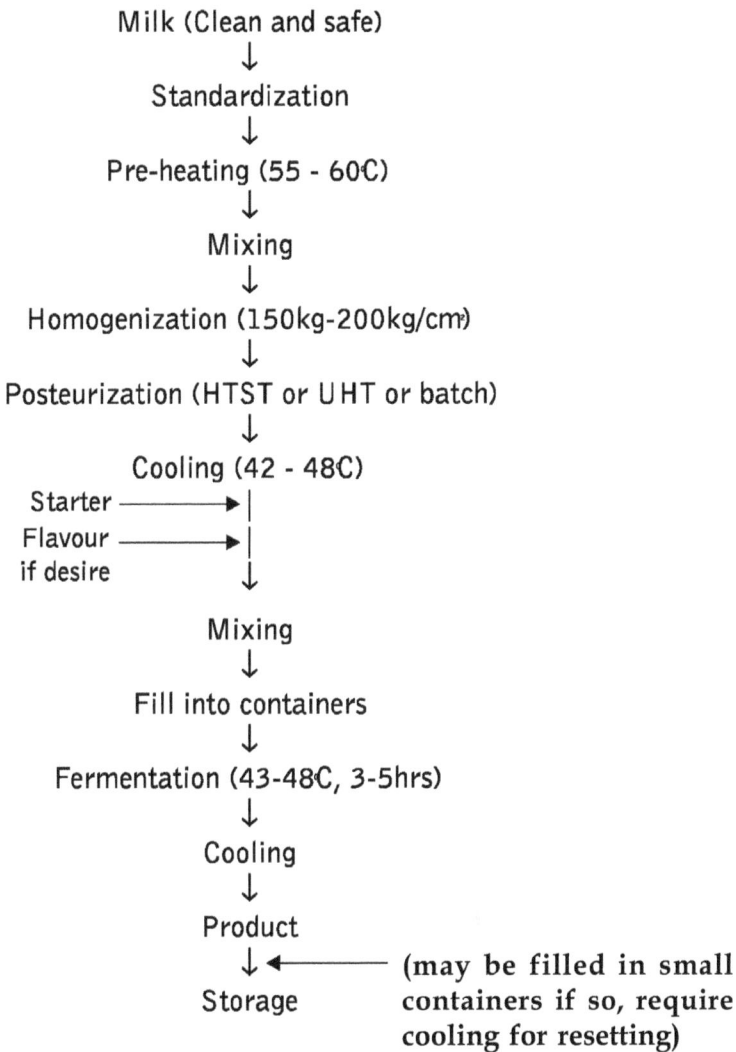

Fig. 3.1: Flow diagram of the production steps of soft or stirred yoghurt.

Milk (Clean and safe)
↓
Standardization
↓ ◄──────── sweetners if required
Pre-heating (55 - 60°C)
↓
Mixing
Stabilizer ──────► ↓
Water ──►↓
Heat to disolve   Mixing
↓
Homogenization (150kg-200kg/cm²)
↓
Posteurization (HTST or UHT or batch)
↓
Cooling (42 - 48°C)
Starter ──────► |
Flavour ──────► |
if desire   ↓
Mixing
↓
Filling into containers
↓
Fermentation (43-48°C, 3-4hrs)
↓
Cooling (5-7°C)
↓
Product (for utilization)
↓
Storage

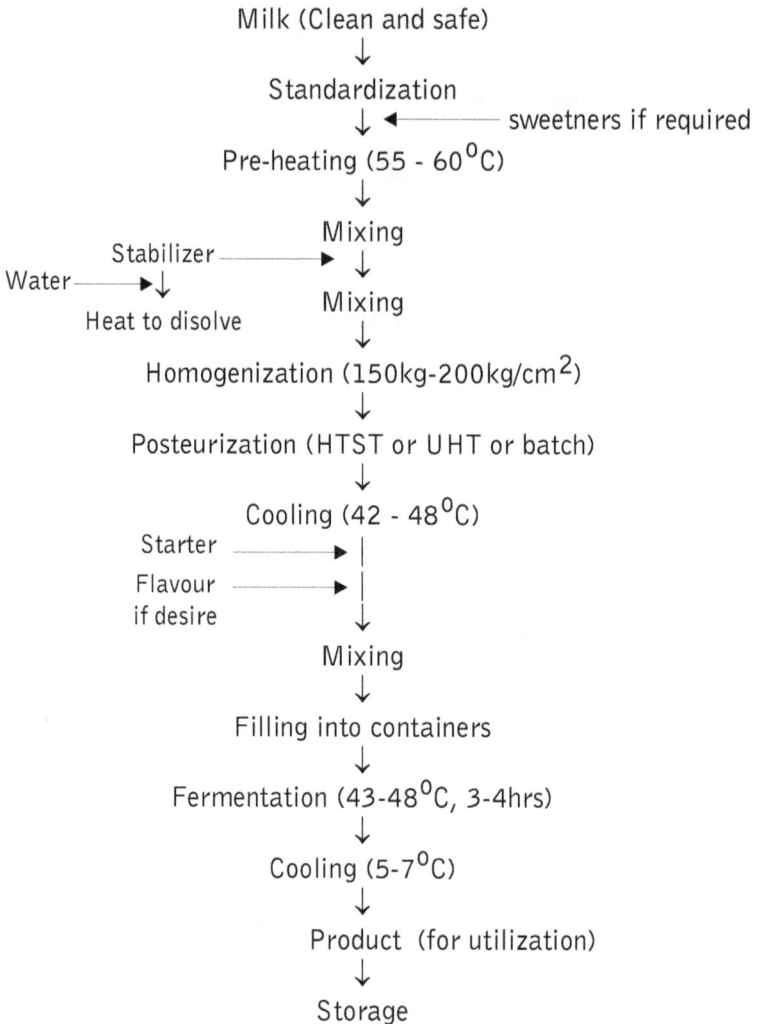

Fig. 3.2: Flow diagram of the production steps of set yoghurt.

Development of microorganism in milk

Specific type of microflora grow better only at specific temperature. The Pseudomonas group (spoilage bacteria) grow best at 10-20°C, but they are capable of growing at 0-5°C whilst other species are not. This type of bacteria is of water born.

Care must be taken during use of water in dairy industry so that this type of problem may not arise. At 10-15°C streptococci and Leuconostoc strat to grow and grow better in the temperature rang of 15-30°C. The streptococci of the lactic group contribute about 90% of the total bacterial population and release acid which is responsible to check the growth of spoilage bacteria. When Pseudomonas group and streptococci grow together at intermediate temperature (15°C), before the release of sufficient acid the flavour of the produce uncleaned flavour due to mixture of different metabolites. At 0.75% acidity the growth of streptococci stops and the slowly growing Lactobacilli continues acid production till 1.5% acid is formed. At this stage when Lactobacilli stop to grow the yeast and moulds will develop in the milk if air is in direct touch with the milk products. Thermophilic streptococci, lactobacilli and aerogenes bacteria may develop at 30-40°C.

In general, most bacteria have an optimum temperature of 15-30°C.

Lactic acid bacteria

Lactic acid starter bacteria is used for the preparation of fermented dairy products. The functional requirement of these bacteria are production of lactic acid after the fermentation of lactose. Also the production of desirable aroma substances, hydrolytic activity towards milk proteins etc. provide safety to the products. General classification of species of lactic acid bacteria for preparation of dairy products are given here under:

Species of dairy lactic acid bacteria

A. Homofermentative lactic streptococci
1. Mesophilic lactococci (growth at 10°C)
    eg. i S. lactis (S.lactis subsp. lactis)
       ii *S.cremoris* (*L.lactis* subsp. cremoris)
       iii *S. lactis* subsp. diacetylactis (*L. lactis* biovar diacetylactis)
2. Thermophilic lactostreptococci (growth at 45-50°C)
    eg. S. Thermophilus

B.   Homofermentative lactobacilli

Group I . Thermobacterium (growth at 45°C) eg.

  i.   Lactobacillus lactis (L.delbrvekii subsp. lactis)

  ii.   L. bulgaricus (L. delbruekii subsp. bulgericus)

  iii. L. acidophilus

  iv.   L. helveticus

Group II. Streptobacterium (growth at 15-45°C)

    eg. L. casei (L.cosei subsp. casei)

C.   Heterofermentative lactic acid bacteria

    eg. Leuconostoc cremoris (L. mesenteroides subsp. cremoris)

For preparation of desired products specific types of bacteria are required. Some of the stairs are more effective in specific conditions whereas, others are not. A good starter culture should have the following criteria:

(i)   Contain selected strains of bacteria/yeast

(ii)   Presence of bacteria in required numbers

(iii) Ratioes of bacteria

(iv)   Survival ability and Viability of bacteria at different stages of products preparation, storage and distribution.

Characteristics of lactic acid bacteria

Lactic acid bacteria are anaerobic, grampositive, to rerate low pH and produce lactic acid. They do not reduce nitrates, do not form spore and can not produce adenosine triphosphate (ATP) by electron transfer (oxidative phosphorelation). They lack porphyrin-cytochrome catalase.

The homofermentative bacteria convert maximum usable corbohydate (upto 85%) to lactic acid, producing 2 mol lactic acid and 2 mol ATP from 1mol monasccharide under specific condition (Fig. 3.3).

LACTOSE
(and GALACTOSE) GLUCOSE GALACTOSE
(medium)

(membrane) PEP PTS PEP PTS permease

(cytoplasm)
LACTOSE-P GALACTOSE
phospho β galactosidase galactokinase
GALACTOSE-1-P

GALACTOSE-6-P GLUCOSE
ATP hexokinase
galactose-6-P isomerase ADP phophoglucomutase
GLUCOSE-6-P GLUCOSE-1-P
glucose phosphate isomerase

TAGATOSE-6-P FRUCTOSE-6-P
ATP ATP
tagatose 6-P kinase phosphofructokinase
ADP ADP
TAGATOSE-1,6-DiP FRUCTOSE-1,6-DiP
tagatose 1,6-P aldolase fructose diphosphate aldolase

DIHYDROXYACETONE-P $\rightleftharpoons$ GLYCERALDEHYDE-3-P
triose phosphate isomerase NAD^+ Pi
3 phosphoglyceraldehyde dehydrogenase
NADH
1,3-DIPHOSPHOGLYCERATE
ADP 3 phosphoglycerate-kinase
ATP
3 PHOSPHOGLYCERATE
phosphoglycerate mutase
2 PHOSPHOGLYCERATE
enolase
PHOSPHOENOLPYRUVATE
ADP
Mg^{++}, K^+ pyruvate kinase + activator
ATP
PYRUVATE
NADH
lactic dehydrogenase
NAD^+
LACTATE

D-TAGATOSE-6-P EMBDEN-MEYERHOF-PARNAS LELOIR
pathway pathway pathway

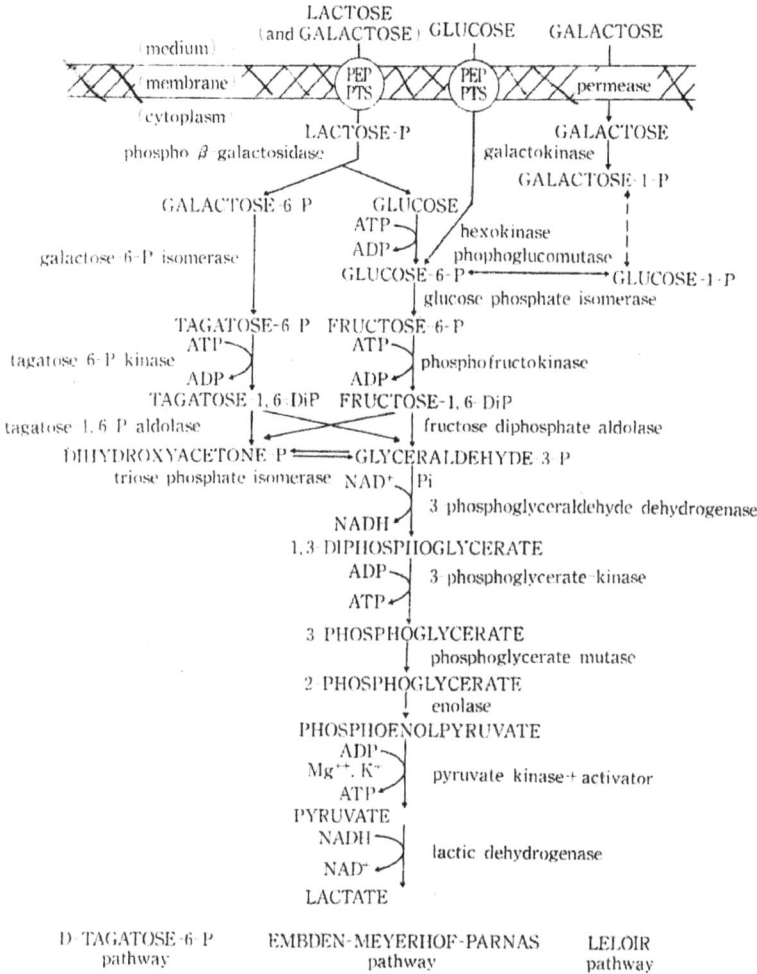

Fig. 3.3: Uptake and metabolism of sugars by homofermentative bacteria.

The heterofermentative lactic acid bacteria produce 1 lactic acid, 1 ethenol including acetic acid, 1 CO_2, 1 ATP (1 ATP from each mol of acetic acid) and small amount of formic acid from 1 monosacchride (Fig. 3.4)

Aerobic metabolism : 1 monosacchride + $6CO_2$ + $6O_2$ + $6H_2O$ + 38 ATP

Chromosomes system is lack in lactic acid bacteria resulting which, NADH produced to harness energy by donation of lectrons from the substrate in the intermediate stage of these systems for sugar catabolism is called out by NADH $\rightarrow$ NAD + reactions linked to substrate electron acceptor reactions to regenerate the NAD + necessary for latter reactions in sugar catabolism.

Few stains of *L.bulgaricus* can utilise some sugars also which is other than lactose, whereas some specific stains of *L.bulgaricus* can only ferment lactose. In aerobic metabolism 1 mole monosacchride produces CO_2, water and energy as:

1 mol monosaccharide + $6O_2$ $\rightarrow$ $6O_2$ + $6H_2O$ + 38 ATP

When galactose is given as an energy source the S.lactis and S. cemoris produce a heterofermentation (Fig. 3.5) forming acetic acid, ethenol, formic acid and lactic acid except S. lactis strains ML8 and S.thermophilus (gal^+).

The growth of S.thermophilus bacteria is better in lactose medium than in media containing glucose or galactose S. lactis utilise glucose and lactose on preferential basis than galactose present in a medium. Permease is specific for galactosides and galactose, and does not lactose or glucose.

Pyruvate is reduced by S. lactis and S. cremoris and formed lactic acid. They also use oxygen dissolved in the medium and release acetic acid, ethenol, acetoin, diacetal and CO_2 from pyruvic acid. Cow milk contains oleic acid which increase the efficiency of pyruvate reduction at pH 5.5 to 6.5 and produce the same as started above except acetic acid. Below pH 5.5 acitic acid production is inhibited.

Lactobacilli produces diacetyl and acetoin from its intracellular pyruvate in the presence of cytric acid or pyruvic acid in absence of oxygen. In normal condition lactobacilli produce only lactic acid when grow on lactose or glucose (Fig. 3.6)

LACTOSE

(medium)

(membrane)

(cytoplasm)

LACTOSE-P

GLUCOSE

ATP

ADP

GALACTOSE 6-P

GLUCOSE 6-P

NAD⁺ ┐ glucose-6-P-dehydrogenase

NADH

D-TAGATOSE-6-P   6-PHOSPHOGLUCONATE

pathway   NAD⁺ ┐

6-phosphogluconate-dehydrogenase

NADH

RIBULOSE-5-P ————— CO₂   NADH,

XYLULOSE-5-P   ┕—— PENTOSE-P pathway → RIBOSE-5-P,

phosphoketolase   NUCLEOTIDE,

GLYCERALDEHYDE-3-P   ACETYL-P ——→ Acetate

NAD⁺ ┐ Pi   CoASH │   ADP   ATP

NADH   ┕ Pi

1,3-DIPHOSPHOGLYCERATE   ACETYL-CoA

ADP ┐   NADH ┐ CoA dependent aldehyde dehydrogenase

ATP ┙   NAD⁺ ┙ CoASH

3-PHOSPHOGLYCERATE   ACETALDEHYDE

2-PHOSPHOGLYCERATE   NADH ┐ alcohol dehydrogenase

NAD⁺ ┙

PHOSPHOENOLPYRUVATE   ETHANOL

ADP ┐

ATP ┙

PYRUVATE

NADH ┐

NAD⁺ ┙

LACTATE

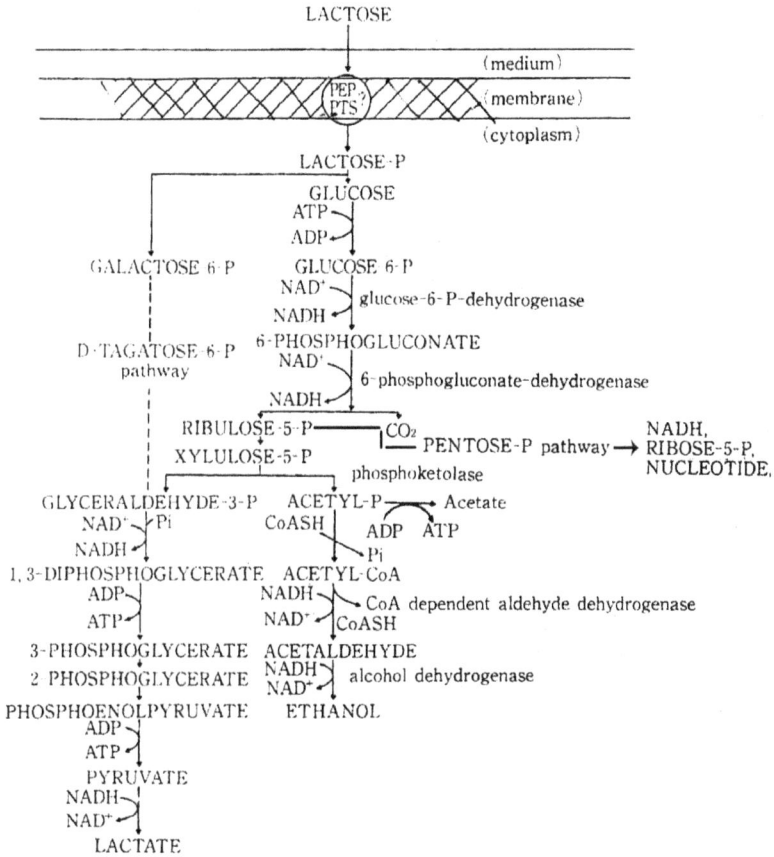

Fig. 3.4: Heterofermentation by *Leuconostoc* app.

D tagatose-6P   Glycolytic   Leloir
  pathway   pathway   pathway

GALACTOSE   GALACTOSE

////// PEP \\\\///////////////// permease //\\\ membrane
////// PTS \\\\///////////////// permease //\\\ membrane
                                                cytoplasm

GALACTOSE-6P   glucose-6P   galactose

tagatose-6P   fructose-6P   GALACTOSE-1P

                                           glucose-1P

TAGATOSE 1,6 diP   FRUCTOSE-1,6-diP

dihydroxyacetone-P ←——→ glyceraldehyde 3P   (A)
                                    NAD'
                                    NADH

                            NADH / NAD'
              (I)   PYRUVATE ←————————→ L (+)-LACTATE
                            lactic
                            dehydrogenase
                    pyruvate
                    formate lyase
                                           acetaldehyde-TPP

FORMATE
                    acetyl CoA
                        NADH
                        NAD⁴

acetaldehyde   acetyl-P
    NADH   ADP
    NAD'   ATP
ETHANOL   ACETATE

A : activation   I : inhibition

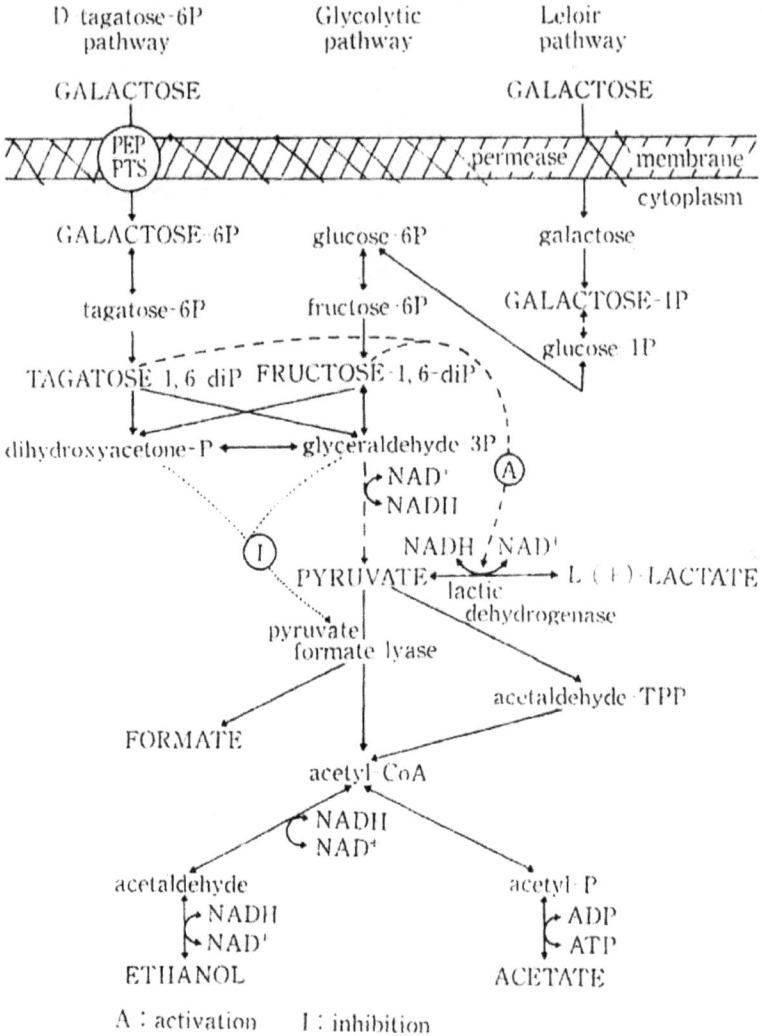

Fig. 3.5: Heterofermentation of galactose in lactococci.

In production of dahi, flavours producing bacteria *leuconostic destranicum* or *L.citrovorous* can also be microporated with mixed or single bacteria of *S. lactis*, *S. cremoris*, *S.diacetilactic*. The flavour in fresh milk is mainly due to diacetyl methyl carbinol

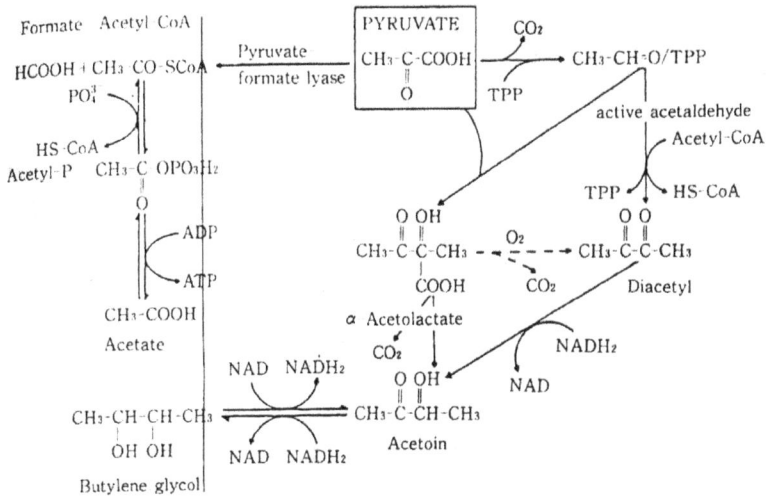

Fig. 3.6: Anaerobic metabolism of pyruvic acid in lactobacilli.

presence in milk (0.018-0.045 ppm). *S.thermophilus* and *L. bulgarieus* can produce maximum of 0.8% acidity in yoghurt. The total tirable acidity in yoghurt in the form of lactic acid should be atleast 0.3per cent in which atleast 0.15% of the total acidity must be obtained by fermentation. During sour dahi preparation *L. bulgaricus* and *S. thermophilus* alongwith other lactic acid bacteria used in sweet dahi can produce upto 1% acidity. The sweet dahi bacteria are *S. lactis,* subsp. *diacetylactis, S. exemoris* and *Leuconostroc* spp. These bacteria can produce upto 0.7% acidity in sweet dahi.

Starter performance factors - These are the following :

1. Rapid growth of bacteria and their ability to develop more acid
2. Fermentation times and temperatures
3. Development of specific flavour, body and texture
4. Survival ability of culture during self life of products
5. Minimise the acid production rate at storage temperature (40-50°F)

6. Helps to enance viscosity (mainly by polysaecharide secreting strains in yoghurt)

7. Works as probiotic properties in the gastrointestinal tract of human beings.

Importance of fermented milk products

1. Acidity helps to develop desired test in milk and milk products.

2. It metabolises lactose and help to reduce lactose intolerance.

3. Increases absorption of minerals in acidic medium (lowering pH).

4. It is resistant to proteolytic enzymes of the gut and helps to reduce decay of body protein which out-go from gut in the form of mucous.

5. Helps to break down potential carcinogenes.

6. It has anagonistic effect against enter-pathogenic bacteria and so supresses the growth of harmful bacteria.

7. During fermentation synthesises vitamin-B which is lost during heat treatment of milk.

8. It help to stimulate bio-immune system.

9. Improves enzymatic/microbial break down of food protien.

10. Lactic acid is useful for the treatment of peptic ulser.

11. Reduces the incidence of intestinal tumors due to its inhibitory effect on mutagenicity of intestinal contents.

12. It improves perilistic movement of the gut and help to remove conspication of stomach.

13. It helps to maintain bile juice production by maintaining serum cholesterol level.

14. It is also helpful in formation of peptides (endogenous and exogenous) from intestinal micriflora. Some of the physiologically active biopeptides thus formed, help to prevent certain diseases.

15. It helps to cure certian skin diseases of the body.

16. In certain cases milk fermenting bacteria may reduce Urea concentration present in milk. The urea may be harmful to some of the useful micro-organisms for their proper growth and development.

17. Some factor in the proto-cooperative between *S. thermophilus* and *L. bulgaricus* in the making of yoghurt seen to be that besides producing formic acid *S. thermoplilus* produces CO_2 from Urea in milk which is useful. Carbondioxide thus produce becomes useful for multiplication of *L. bulgarieus*.

18. Lactic acid is an energy for heart, respiratory organs, and is also useful in skeletal muscle, kidney, liver and brain, etc.

19. During proteolysis aroma compound acetaldehyde is developed from threonine in the yoghurt.

4 Quality Control

During handling of milk and milk products at different steps of processing, manufacturing, storage and distribution quality assurance/quality control is most essential. The quality assurance denotes the strategic management function that establishes policies related to quality, adopt programes to meet the established goals, and be assured and provide confidence for its application. Quality control is a tactical fuction that carries out those programes identified by quality assurance to be necessary to teach the quality goals.

According to the International standard Organisation (ISO) quality is "The totality of functions and characteristics of products or service that bear on its ability to satisfy steated or implied needs quality incompasses safety, hygiene, reliability, wholesomeness, acceptance by consumer and quality conveys different meanings to different people."

A product like guava jam of the same quality is prepard by different factories in the country and abrod but a few of them are like very much by most of the consumers. In the same way reliability of the product, credit of the brand/organisor also help to make the products more popular.

According to Wakhlu (1995) the total quality can be defined as "Performance superiority in delighting customers. The means used are people, committed to employing organizational resources to provide value to consumers, by doing the right things right the first time, every time."

QUALITY : THE INTERNATIONAL CHALLENGES (Khanna, 2001)

From the industrial point of view, there are many compulsions to produce 'Quality' milk and milk products. These are :

- In 1991 the economic policy was liberalized : to allow for more foreingn investment, by removal of many trade restrictions, by removing many restrictions on imports and exports, and creation of free trade zones. This moved the Indian dairy sector to the freshold of intense international competition and globalization. For example, now all dairy products can be imported and exported without any restrictions.

- As a member and signatory to the World Trade Organization, India is committed to reduce the custom duty to 25% or less, reduce all types of subsidies to 10% or less. These are of course guarded as long as the balance of payment status does not favour India.

- A preliminary analysis, however, indicated (Bhasin, 1995) that WTO conditionalities favoured the Indian dairy industry and opened up opportunities for export of dairy products.

- At present 85% of the dairy products in the world export market are from the US, the EC, New Zealand and Australia. Comparatively, the exports from India are negligible. The Gujarat Co-operative Milk Marketing Federation is the largest exporter of dairy products from India for the last five consecutive years, and during 1997-98 their exports were Rs. 26 Crores for butter, ghee, shrikhand and gulabjamuns to the USA, New Zealand, Singapore, Thailand and Iraq (GCMMF Annual Report 1997-98, 1998-99).

- With the World Trade Organization working towards elimination of quotas, lowering of custom tariffs, diminishing government subsidies, converting non-tariff measures into tarrifs and increasing the transparency in national legislations, the world is emerging as a single market place (for dairy products).

- The WTO agreement on application of Sanitary and Phytosanitary Measures (SPS) require that these measures be based on scientific principles. While countries are encouraged to use international standards, allowance is made for implementing measures stricter than the international standards.

- The WTO aggreement on Technical Barriers to Trade (TBT) provides that all WTO members must refrain from adopting such standards as discriminate against import of products by creating unnecessary obstacles to the international trade.

- With regard to food safety measures SPS requires that national standards be harmonized with international standards, guidelines and recommendations adopted by the Codex Alimentarius Commission (CAC). For the dairy sector the CAC guidelines are based on the recommendations of the following international panels:

- CCMMP : Codex Committee on Milk and Milk Products
- CCFAC : Codex Committee on Food Additives and Contaminants
- CCPR   : Codex Committee on Pesticide Residues
- CCRVDF : Codex Committee on Residues of Veterinary Drugs in Food
- CCFL   : Codex Committee on Food Labeling
- CCFH   : Codex Committee on Food Import and Export Inspection and Certification Systems
- CCMA   : Codex Committee on Method of Analysis and Sampling
- JECFA : Joint FAO/WHO Expert Committee on Food Additives
- JMPR   : Joint FAO/WHO Meeting on Pesticide Residues.

Food Hazards

The main hazards of foods are the following:

(i)   Microbiological danger

(ii)   Chemicals contamination

(iii) Contamination of extraneous (foreign) matters.

Milk and milk products must be free from the microorganisms like clostridium botulium, clostridium prefringens, salmonella, staphylococcus aureus, camphylobacter jejuni, Listeria monocytogenes, Escherichia coli, yersinia enterocolitica and molds. Molds produce micotoxins which is more toxic for humans

The residues of the drugs given to the animals are present in the milk. Some harmful chemicals like BHC, DDT, 2-4D etc enters in the animal body through feeds and fodders. Heavy metals, chlorine, acid sanitizers etc. are also dangerous for health of the humans.

Dirt, soil paints, metal filings, wooden splinters, oils etc. may enters into the products during processing which may affects the flavour, colour and chemical quality of the milk.

General symptoms of microbial toxins in the body:

Nausea, stomach ache, vomiting, diarrhoea, sudden weakness, dryness on lips surface, fever, difficulties in breathing and swallowing etc.

Hazard Analysis and Critical control Points (HACCP)

Milk and milk products should be acceptable and also safe to the consumers. Aiming to these, in recent advancement, the manufacturing defects in foods are reduced through the use of Good Manufacturing Practices (GMPs) in processing, inspections and laboratory analysis of finished products/packaged products to ensure their specifications under quality assurance. The Hazard Analysis and Critical Control Points (HACCP) is an integral part of the total quality system (TQS) or total quality management (TQM).

HACCP is a system which identifies, evaluates and controls hazards which are singificant for food safety. The Critical Control Point (CCP) is a step in the process at which control can be applied and is essential to prevent or eliminate a food safety hazard or reduce it to an acceptable level. In the hazard analysis Critical limit is a critarian which separate acceptability from unacceptability. HACCP system was developed for assuring safety of the low acid canned food. Risk analysis is a process which comprises risk assessment, risk management and risk communication (FAO/WHO Report, 1995,1997).*

FAO/WHO joint expert consultation report on application of Risk Management to Food Safety Matters, 1997.

The principle for HACCP involves two main points :

(i)   Hazard Analysis - This involves a critical examination at all the manufactureing steps/processes of foods for above three hazards.

(ii) Critical Control Point - A point where maximum possibility of the hazards may occurs during processing and may cause spoilege of finished products. Critical control required the following range of measure should be established for the CCP:

    (i)   Critical limits (location of Crital point & its parameter)

    (ii) Monitoring system parameter procedure for each parameter

    (iii) Corrective action if the control is unacceptable

    (iv) Documentation and record keeping frequent of monitoring indicate more acuracy

    (v)   Verification procedures (criteria for deciding acceptable & Unacceptable levels)

The united state National Advisory Committee on Microbiological Criteria of Food (NACMCF) given seven principles of the HACCPs which are as follows:

(i)   Conduct a harzard analysis and risk assessment

(ii) Determin the critical control points (including CCP, and CCP2)

(iii) Establish critical limites (Specifications for each CCP)

(iv) Monitor each CCP

(v)   Establish corrective action to be taken if a deviation occurs at a CCP

(vi) Establish a record-keepong system, and

(vii) Establish verification procedures

Benefits of HACCP

1. A preventive approach to food packaging safety

2. Can help identify process improvements

3. Reduce the need for and the cost of end product testing

4. Is complementary to quality measurement systems such as ISO: 9000

5. Provide evidence of due diligence

6. Reduces the likelihood of product recall and adverse publicity

7. Enhances customers satisfaction and reduces dissatisfaction

8. Facilities better understanding of food packaging safety issues throughout the organisation

9. Improves staff morale and motivation through a cleaner working environment

10. Improves staff performance through the promotion of team spirit

11. Help maintain in compliance to the BRC Global standard-Food Packaging

Total Quality Management (TQM) - It is a Japanese technique. The Managing Director of the largest dairy organization - GCMMF in India feels that there is nothing Japanese or Western about TQM. Vyas (1999) said that the basic priniciples of TQM are universal, fundamental and commonsensical. The funtional principles of TQM are here under.

1. Customer Orientation- Customer is all for flourising any type of business. Therefore, it is issential to identify the proper customers, understand their requirements and measure customers satisfaction.

2. Maintain quality for customers satisfaction.

3. Make Contineous improvement of quality.

4. Improve communication process from organization to customers

5. Educate the employees through organizing training for improvement in their areas of weakness to help them for imporving their efficiency.

6. The goal and quality indicator should be recorded and make it measurable. This will help in setting standards, judging tolerence limits of critical points and establish the process to produce the products of predetermined quality standards.

7. All the practices mentioned must be done together, nothing can be achieved through isolation

Meeting the challenges of quality

Total Quality management became the fore most requirement of any organization involved in the quality production in the world. This is followed parallel with the normal functioning of the organization. The organizations should follow the following steps:

(a) Identify with ISO (International Standards Organization)

The category of organization fit in the following ISO should follow the standard:

(i) ISO : 9001 - a standard that provides a model for quality assurance in desing/development, production and installation and servicing.

(ii) ISO: 9002 - a standard that provides a model for quality assurance in production and installation.

(iii) ISO : 9003 - a standard that provides a model for quality assurance in final inspection and test.

ISO: 9002 and ISO : 9003 are subsets of ISO : 9001. For dairy industry ISO : 9002 is sufficient. These all should be implemented with the GHP, GMP and HACCP.

(b) Hygienec Practices - To ensure the safety of the products it is necessary to reduce the introduction/occurance of hazard at different stages of production.

(c) Good House keeping - It is the prime responsibility of the person/s involve to the place of work. The principles of house keeping - 'SCAPS' or '5S' are summarised below:

1. 'S' SORTING OUT (Selri) - Separate the items of use from not needed on daily basis.

2. 'C' CLEANING (Seiso) - Seiso refers to cleaning the work place and the instruments by our selves, and not depend on others to clean.

3. 'A' ARRANGEMENT (Section) - All the items should be properly identified labeled and Kept at its predecided place.

4. 'P' PERSONAL HYGIENE (Seiketsu) - Persons involved at the place should maintain personal hygiene and cleanliness around his/her work place.

5. 'S' SELF DISCIPLINE (SHITSUKE) - Every one should be disciplined to follow the rules without compromise with any thing during working. Puntuality, devotion, honesty etc. make the persons disciplined.

(d) Adoptation of good manufacturing practices

This includes the condition of the surroundings where buildings of the factory is situated design of the buildings, lighting and ventilcation arrangement type and durability of building materials, protection from unwanted elements (animals, birds, insects etc.).

(e)   Maintaining HACCP and TQM at the organisation.

BIS Standards for dahi and yoghurt

1.   Titrable acidity (max) 0.7% sour 1%

2.   Coliform count < 10/g

3.   Yeast and mould count < 100/g

4.   Phosphatase test   - ve

Table. 1 : Score card for dahi and yoghurt

S.No.	Items	Perfect Score
1.	Flavour	45
2.	Body & Texture	30
3.	Acidity	15
4.	Colour & appearance	5
5.	Packaging	5

(Yoghurt score card by Nelson & Trout, 1964)

5 Packaging System of Food

Packaging is a means of ensuring the safe delivery of the product from production unit to consumer in sound condition at the chipest cost. The following stages may be the most efficient points :

1. Production
2. Logistics
3. Sales
4. Consumption
5. Disposal - a minimum ecological problem.

Purpose

1. It should be suitable for the products.
2. It fulfills the logistics requirements for production and their distribution.
3. Efficient to attained the best sales-effect of the product.
4. It may fulfill the best interest in the consumers.

Function of Packaging

1. To hold the contents.
2. Protect the contents against hazzards.
3. Ability to perform better for high speed filling, cleaning and collecting in shortest time.
4. Identify the product and guide about the handling during transportation.
5. Convenient through the production, storage and distribution.

Criteria to judge the packaging : Nine words used in PACKAGING denotes the following:

P. Prevention   -   to prevent the content from hazzards.

A. Available   -   it should be easily available.

C. Cheaper   -   materials should be cheaper.

K. Keeping quality   -   it has good protection ability and longer life.

A. Adoptable   -   it should be easy to adapt and handle.

G. Gallant/Glace   -   it should be attractive to consumers.

I. Imparmanent   -   it should be easy to disposed off without harm to environment.

N. Nativeness   -   it should have their natural/original property during storage and distribution.

G. Governability   -   it should be gustless but not graveolence.

During advertising of a product the following factors may influence the success of a package (Head and steward, 1989):
1.   Standout
2.   Content identification
3.   Imagery
4.   Distintiveness
5.   Adaptability
6.   Suitability
7.   Legalety

During storage of a product the following main factors are responsible for deterioration:
1.   Light - During display of contents light transmission is required but it should be restricted to product which are

susceptible to spoilage by light i.e. lipid, riboflavin, natural pigments etc.

2. Heat - The material must have ability to with stand the processing conditions without interaction of the contents and without damage the materials.

3. Moisture - Moisture exchange control is necessary to prevent microbial and engymatic spoilages, softening or drying out of products.

Forms of packaging materials

Earlier dahi and ghee was protected and transperted from one place to other place in earthen pots. But it is unhyigenic and not durable. wooden basket and drums were also in practice. At present the following packaging materials are in practice:

1. Tin containers

2. Aluminium boil

3. Glass - jars and bottles

4. Paper - Coloured, coated with wax, glass line etc.

5. Paper Board - Pulp, duplex, triplex (grease, corrugated, moulded etc).

6. Plastic/metals - application in thin flim/layers. It may be of different types:

    a. Low Density Polyethylene (LDPE)

    b. Linear Low Density Polyethylene (LLDPE)

    c. High Density Polyethylene (HDPE)

    d. High molecular High Density Polyethylene (HMHDP)

    e. Biaxially oriented polypropyline (BOPP) films

    f. Polyethylene terephthalate (PET) films

    g. Metallized polypropylene (MPP) films

    h. Metallized polyester (MPET) films

Indian standards for packaging of milk and milk products are given in table - 1

In modifide atmosphere packaging (MAP) most of the pack are constracted from four basic polymers:

1.   Poly vinyl chloride (PVC)
2.   Poly ethylene terephthalate (PET)
3.   Polypropylene (PP)
4.   Polyethylene (PE)

Table. 1   :   Indian standards for packaging of milk and milk
              products

Metallic Packaging	
IS 8221 :	1976 Code of practice for corrosion prevention of metals and components in package, Reaffirmed 1990
Tin Packaging	
IS 4079 :	1976 Canned Rasogolla
IS 9991 :	1981 Condensed milk cans, Reaffirmed 1992
IS 10339 :	1988 Ghee, Vanaspati and edible oil tins (1st revision) (Amendment 1) Reaffirmed 1994
Aluminium Foil Packaging	
IS 3603 :	1978 Paper aluminium foil laminates for general packaging. Reaffirmed 1989
IS 8970 :	1991 Aluminium foil laminates for packaging (1st revision)
Aluminium Bottles	
IS 3603 :	1988 Seamless aluminium bottles (1st revision)
Plastic Film Packaging	
IS 7019 :	Glossary of terms in plastic and flexible packaging excluding paper (2nd revision)
IS 10171 :	1987 Guide on suitability of plastics for food packaging
Polyethylene/ Flexible Packaging	
IS 11824 :	1986 Paper coated high density polyethylene woven sacks for packing skim milk powder
IS 14129 :	1994 Flexible packaging materials for packing of Vanaspati in 10kg & 15 kg packs
IS 10840 :	1994 Blow moulded HDPE containers for packing of Vanaspati-specifications
IS 11352 :	1994 Flexible packaging materials for packing of Vanaspati in 100 gm, 200 gm, 500 gm, 1 kg, 2 kg, & 5 kg, packs

Paper/ Fiberboard Packaging		
IS 3263	:	1981 Waxed paper for confectionery (1st revision). Reaffirmed 1998
IS 3962	:	1976 Waxed paper for general packaging (Amendment 1), Reaffirmed 1996
IS 4261	:	1967 Glossary of terms relating to paper & pulp based packaging materials (Amendments 2)
IS 7162	:	1973 Glossary of terms relating to paper & flexible packaging
IS 9313	:	1979 Corrugated fibreboard boxes for export packaging of glass jars & bottles filled with processed foods
IS 9988	:	1981 Waxed paper for bread & biscuit, Reaffirmed 1993
IS 10177	:	1982 Ice cream cups & lips, Reaffirmed 1993
IS 12212	:	1987 Corrugated fibreboard boxes for transprot packaging of butter packed in primary carton
Glass Bottles		
IS 1392	:	1983 Glass milk bottles (3rd revision). Reaffirmed 1998
IS 6654	:	1992 Glass containers : Glossary of terms (2nd revision), Reaffirmed 1998
Milk Bottles		
IS 1613	:	1960 Milk bottle crates (Amendment 1)
General Packaging Code		
IS 10106 (Part - I/Sec 2) :		1990 Packaging code : Part I Product packaging, Sec 1 Foodstuffs & perishables
Some guidelines for use of plastic materials have also been published:		
IS 2798 Methods of test for plastic containers (1st revision)		
IS 8747	:	1997 Methods of test for environmental stress-crack resistance of blow-moluded polyethylene containers
IS 9883	:	1981 List of pigments and colorants for use in plastics in contact with foodstuffs, pharmaceuticals and drinking water
IS 10171	:	1987 Guide on suitability of plastics for food packaging

Reasons for use of plastics for packaging :

1. Plastic are very light in weight.
2. They are very flexible and can be given any shape.
3. They are resistant to moisture.
4. They can be clean easily.
5. They do not break easily.
6. Broken pieces are not harmful as compared to metals and glass.
7. Oxygen, gases and moisture can not come in contact with the products as they works as barrier properties.
8. They are transferable similar to glass, whereas metals paper board are not performing the same.
9. They do not develop off-flavour.
10. They can be sterilized by conventional method.
12. They are easy in sealing.
13. Very less amount of materials can be packed by plastics.
14. They can be disposed off easily without adverse ecological effect.

Modified Atmosphere Packaging (MAP)

Modified Atmosphere Packaging (MAP) is also called as controlled Atmosphere Packaging (CAP). In this process atmosphere air present inside the sealed package is replaced by known gas or some known mixture of gases. This replacement of air is done to regulate the environment inside the package. Carbon dioxide, Oxygen, nitrogen and water vapour are mainly regulated the atmosphere of inside the package.

Oxygen (O_2)

Oxygen inhibits the growth of strictly anaerobic bacteria wheras, stimulates the growth of aerobic bacteria . To preserve the fresh red meat O_2 is essential for maintaining the pigment (myoglobin to oxymyoglobin). In MAP method meat is packed in an 80% O_2 and 20% CO_2. In fatty fish it may cause oxidative rencidity and in cured meat colour problems are exhist. Under this circumstances atmosphere packaging 35% CO_2 and 65% N_2 are used.

Nitrogen (N_2)

N_2 is an inert and tasteless gas. It is less soluble in fat and water both. N2 is mainly used to delay oxidative rancidity and check the growth of aerobic microrganisms. This gas is used to displace O_2 in the packs.

Carbon dioxide (CO_2)

Carbon dioxide is soluble in water and fat both. In modified atmosphere, the overall effect on microorganisms is an extension of the log phase of growth and decrease in the growth rate during the logarithmic growth phase. In the presence of 1007. CO_2 in the pack reduced significantly the concentration of O_2 in the MAP resulting which product seperation in cream, increased drip in fresh meat, discolouration, physiological damage to vegetables and fruit are observed. These adverse effects are mainly due to the low levels of oxygen rather than CO_2.

Other gases

SO_2, N_2O (nitrous oxide), NO (nitric oxide), H_2, He, Ne, Cl_2, Ozone etc, are also used. But it is limited by safety concerned, legislation, negative effects on the organolaptic properties, cost and adverse consumers response of packaged products.

Aseptic packaging :

In this process milk and milk products after sterilization or ultra high temperature (UHT) processing are filled under asefitic conditions in multi-layer high barrier packages. The self life of the materials enhanced upto 6 months at room temperature (20-30°C). This depends mainly on the composition and pretreatment of the products, type of packaging materials and packaging system.

Packages used in aseptic packaging :

(a)　Flexible laminates - Retort pouch

(b)　Rigid laminates -

　　　Tetra Brik system

　　　Liqui - Pak system

　　　Gasti DOG system

　　　Conofast system

　　　Combiblock system

　　　Starasept system

(In this system cartons, roll stock (Web) or preformed plastic tubes like materials are used)

　　　Bag in box system

　　　Steriglen system

Pack design and packaging equipment

Mainly three basic retail MAP forms are :

1.　Semi-rigid tray-for meat

2.　The pillow pouch formate-for fresh salad

3.　The flowpack formate - for cheese and bakery products

Some times in retail formats 'master pack', 'mother pack' and 'bag in box' are also used, which allow centralized packaging operations.

For these packs four types of machinary are used :

1.　Rigid and semi-rigid tray packers

2.　Flexible horizontal flow wrap packers

3.　Flexible verticle form-fill seal packers

4.　Bulk box/drum packers

Tin can Filling Machine

This is used for filling ghee into open top container of 1,2 and 5 kg size. The ghee contact surfaces of machine are made from

AISI-304 stainless steel. All the pipe are SMS standards. The loading frame is covered with stainless steel. The capasity of this machine by manually operated is 10-12 tins/minute and by autometic operation 50 tins/minute.

Form-fill and seal (FFS) Machine

This machine is used for packaging products in plastic containers, plastic/alminium foil coated board. Dahi, shrikhand, lassi and ghee are common for packaging by this machine. Ghee is generally packed in 500 ml or 1000 ml pouches whereas others in 200 to 500 ml.

By ghee pouch FFS machine pillow type pouches are formed, filled and sealed. 500 ml and 1000 ml ghee are packed in one operation. Nearly 1000 pouches of ghee are pack/hour.

Multi-fill packaging machine :

This machine has seperate container conveyor on horigontal plane with a elevated product conveyer to the filling hopper. This can be used for packing all the indigenous sweets, vegetable fruit, instant quick frozen (IQF) products in various shape and size of plastic container with thermo sealed foil or lid.

Vacuum and gas packaging machine

For mechanical air replacement gas flushing and compressed vaccum techniques are used. In gas filling method, gas is injected in the package to replace air and sealed. The air present inside the pack is diluted and resulting which the oxygen level comes to 2 to 5%. In compressed vacuum method a desired gas mixture is injected inside the package only after evacuation of air. The nozzle and chamber types vacuum packaging machines are used for this purpose. Whole milk powder, bady food, resogolla, gulabjamun etc. are packed by this machine.

Advantage of MAP technology

1. Dairy, fish, meat and poultry products can be packed in same manner.
2. All round visibility and clear view of the product is improved.

3. Hygeinic sealed product is free from product drip and odour.
4. The chances of growth of pathogenes are very negligible even in long period of storage.
5. Packed product can be stored for longer duration (by 50 to 400 times) without the loss of its quality.
6. The storage cost of the product is reduced due to better utilization of labour, equipments and space.

Disadvantages of MAP technology

1. Capital cost of gas, packaging materials and packaging machinary are involved.
2. Pack volume increased resulting which transportation cost increases.
3. Temperature controlled storage facility is needed failing which food borne pathogenes may grow during the storage.

6 Works Imported on Yoghurt

Amongst several varieties of fermented milk and milk products, yoghurt is the most popular with different names in the world. In India, yoghurt known for its typical flavour, is the only variety manufactured in substantial quanities. Yoghurt is usually made from cow milk. In view of increasing demand for yoghurt, there is a need to find out a suitable technology or method for the manufacture of good quality yoghurt using standardized cow and buffalo milk with enhanced flavour, suitable body and texture, colour and appearance, acidity etc. This project has been taken up aiming to develope a good quality yoghurt from cow and buffalo milk by standardizing the milk with different level of fat, SNF, bacterial composition and incubation temperature and by finding out their effect on physical attributes (flavour, body and texture, colour and appearance, acidity etc.) and chemical composition. The work carried out by different workers in India and abroad earlier related to this project is reviewed here, under following heads (Kumar. 2002):

2.1 Effect of milk on physico-chemical quality of yoghurt

2.2 Effect of fat and SNF on physico-chemical quality of yoghurt

2.3 Effect of starter culture (ratio of rods and cocci) and incubation temperature on physico-chemical quality of yoghurt.

2.4 Effect of feeding yoghurt on growth rate and feed efficiency, blood profile in rats.

2.1 Effect of Milk on a Physico-chemical Quality of Yoghurt

When 16 h milk cultured with *Streptococcus thermophilus* and/or *Lactobacillus bulgaricus* were incubated at 37°C in sterilized (100°C for 30 min) fresh cow's or buffalo's milk, the mixed culture of the two organisms developed higher acidity and produced more volatile acid and acetaldehyde than did either organism alone, but proteolytic activity was lower than that of *L. bulgaricus* alone (Khanna and Singh, 1979). All cultures developed more volatile acidity production in buffalo's than in cow's milk. The greater acid production by the mixed culture was due to enhance growth of streptococci. The growth of *L.bulgaricus* in mixed culture was less vigourus than in pure culture in both types of milk.

Alm (1982) investigated total lactic acid and relative amounts of L(+) and D(-) lactic acid in cultured milk products. The products were regular milk cultured butter milk (filmyolk), yoghurt, kafir, ropy milk (langmojolk), UHT low fat milk (lattmjolk), low fat acidophilus milk, V-medium, acidophilus milk and bifidus milk. Amount of total lactic in the cultured products was in the same range (0.6-1.2%) as for lactic acid in products from other countries. In all products L(+) lactic acid was the major isomer formed. Of the total lactic acid, 0-10 and approximate 40% was of D(-) configuration in respective acidophilus milk and yoghurt.

The triglyceride composition of yoghurt made from cow's, ewe's and goat's milk was not significantly differ from that of unfermented milk (Baccignone et al., 1982). Yoghurt made from cow milk contained more free caprylic, caproic, lauric and linolenic acids, yoghurts from ewe milk contained more free palmitic, stearic and oleic acids and yoghurt from goat milk contained more free caproic, caprylic, palmitoleic acids.

Singh and Kaul (1982) reported the buffalo milk yoghurt showed to have higher organo-leptic scores. The cultures grown in buffalo milk produced more acidity and had higher proteolytic acitivty than cultures grown in cow and goat's milk.

Al-Dahhan (1984) studied the effect of different kinds of milk on quality of laben. Experimental laben made with *Streptococcus lactis*/*Lactobacillus bulgaricus* starter from the following milks had fat, protein and T.S. content respectively, as follows

(i) Cow's milk + dried skim milk - 3.46, 3.87 and 15.88% (ii) Cow's milk -3.42, 3.04 and 12.27% (iii) Ewe's milk - 4.26, 6.18 and 15.81% (iv) goat's milk - 3.66, 4.0 and 13.57% (v) cow's +goat's milk (50% v/v) milk - 3.52, 3.52 and 13.18 per cent. He noted that flavour scores increased ($P < 0.01$) during storage and at 6 days score were the highest (44) for laben made with (iii) and lowest (42.52 and 41.81) for laben made with (iv) and (vi) respectively. Body and texture score of different labens varied considerably ($P < 0.01$) and were the highest (29.62 and 28.3 at 1 days) in laben made with (iii) also had the highest acidity (1.43, 1.58 and 1.65% lactic acid at 1,4 and 6 days respectively).

Chopra et al. (1984) prepared a yoghurt like product from soya milk alone and after adding 10, 20 or 30% skim milk. Soya milk supplemented with 1% sucrose (w/v) was incubated with individual or mixed cultures of Sterptococcus thermophilus and Lactobacillus acidophilus and growth was examined over a 16 h period. Results showed that mixed cultures produced more acid than single culture, addition of skim milk further enhanced acid production. Sensory evaluation revealed the absence of beany flavour in all the products, mixed cultures gave a better product than single cultures. Incorporation of skim milk upto 20% enchaced acceptability, but > 20% weakened the body of the products.

Reconstituted whole cow's milk, evaporated milk, condensed milk, goat milk and yoghurt contained 2.6%, 7.4%, 3.8%, 3.5% and 2.4% fat, 3.2%, 6.9%, 8.1%, 3.5% crude protein and 5.27%, 9.2%, 66.0%, 5.0% and 3.8 per cent carbohydrates (Abreu et al., 1985). Dahi made from milk of Jersy X Haryana crosses contained 4.8% fat, 3.41% protein. 4.7% lactose, 0.70% ash, 2.8% casein and 13.6% total solids (Sanyal and Yadav, 1986). They have also reported that product had better appearance, body and texture than dahi made from milk of Brown Swiss x Haryana or Holstein -Friesian x Haryana cross breds.

Manjunath and Abraham (1986) made yoghurt from goat's milk adjusted to 15% TS by adding cow's dried skim milk. When it compared with cow's milk yoghurt, goat's milk yoghurt showed an increased rate of lactic acid production and decreased rate of acetaldehyde production. Proteolytic activity was similar for both yoghurt. Goat milk yoghurt had a softer body, whiter in colour, and less wheying off properties. Member's of task panel could not distinguish between the two yoghurts for flavour and taste.

Brendchag (1987) reported that the yoghurt gel structure depends on the types of milk used, its microbiological quality and composition mainly. He found that increasing yoghurt T.S. from 12-20% resulted in a densed gel structure with more casein micelles and fewer smaller spores. TS of < 16% gave yoghurt with a good gel structure.

Kehagias et al. (1987) detected that the ewe's milk yoghurt had the highest penetration and viscosity, lowest volume of serum and had a better flavour than goat's milk yoghurt. Penetration force and vicosity of indigenous goat milk yoghurt were higher and serum separated that yoghurt made from goat's milk is not more significantly rated to cow's milk yoghurt, taste pannel preferred yoghurt made from cow's milk.

The quality of yoghurt made from fresh skim milk and fortified with skim powder was examined by Resubal et al. (1987). They standaridized the skim milk to (i) 14, (ii) 17 and (iii) 20% TS using dried skim milk and used to make yoghurt and stored it upto 20 days at 5-100C. Finally, they found the scores for taste, odour, consistency and acceptability (max) were 7.04, 7.32, 7.41 and 7.00 for control yoghurt (made from whole milk 20% TS), 6.36, 6.81, 5.49 and 5.73 for (i), 6.83, 7.48, 7.66 and 7.28 for (ii) and 7.21, 7.48, 7.66 and 7.33 for (iii) respectively. Age of yoghurt did not significantly affect on sensory quality (atributes) for all yoghurt. Samples stored for 5, 15 and 20 days showed highest scores for taste. Values for lactic acid and pH respectively were 1.4% and 4.19 for control, 1.43% and 4.26 for (i), 1.32% and 4.14 for (ii) 1.21 and 4.00 for (iii) Lactic acid content increased and pH correspondingly decreased on storage.

Kehagias et. al. (1989) studied the composition of set type yoghurt in relation to its physical properties, made from indigenous saanen and saanen cross breds and found that penetration force and viscosity of yoghurt showed good correlation with Ca and fat content. Milk from indigenous breeds had the highest concentration of TS, protein, fat and Ca and yoghurt prepated from it had the highest instron pentration force and viscosity. Organoleptically yoghurt prepared from saanen goat milk was least preferred, while yoghurt from indigenous breeds approched, in preference, commercial brands of yoghurt from cow milks. Physical characteristics of yoghurt were improved by increasing SNF contents and by adding commercially available cow milk proteins, while by increasing fat content and adding $CaCl_2$, physical characteristics of yoghurt were not improved, despite the good correlation between fat and Ca content of goat milk and penetration force and viscosity of yoghurt.

Yoghurt made from buffalo milk (6.3% fat and 4.73% protein) was most acceptable when milk was pastuirized at 75°C for 5 min. (Cardoso Castaned, et. al., 1991). Average chemical composition of milk, fat, protein, TS and acidity were 6.1, 4.68, 16.66, 1.0 percent, respectively.

The yoghurt made from buffalo skim milk at different heat treatments and holding time (75° C/ 5min, 85° C/10 min and 95° C/15 min) was significantly affected (P < 0.05) by pasteurization temperature but holding time and heat treatment of 85° C/5 min. was considered adequate for buffalo milk to be used in yoghurt manufacture (Iniguez et. al., 1991). Yoghurt manufactured from this milk contained 0.1% fat, 4.65% protein, 9.77% TS, 4.33% lactose, 0.69% mineral and 1.01% acidity.

Tamime et. al. (1991) made two types of labneh from cow and goat or ewe milk by (a) traditional style - labneh was produced by straining yoghurt in cloth bag and (b) UF- labneh was produced by UF of warm yoghurt and a portion of all products homogenized by a lactic acid homogenizer, and reported that homogenization markedly decreased firmness of goat and ewe milk labneh, and is therefore not recommended in industrial production and firmness of labneh made form cow milk was affected by homogenization to lesser extent. The labneh samples contained 20.5-22.5% TS, 6.7 - 8.2% protein and 7.8 - 8.9% fat.

Ahmed (1992) manufactured zabadi from fresh cow or goat milk with or without addition of 5 or 10% skim milk powder (SMP) and found that the zabadi made from cow or goat milk supplemented with SMP had lower pH and higher acidity than made form milk without SMP. Addition of 5% SMP greatly improved the quality of zabadi produced from cow milk, while quality of the zabadi made from goat milk was improved when 10% SMP was added.

Noeman and Shalaby (1992) studied the effect of culturing on the nutritional value of milk. For this, they made two types of fermented milk product from buffalo milk viz., zabadi and acidophilus (semi-skim milk containing 3% fat). Result showed, culturing caused considerable alteration in chemical composition of these two products. Lactose content decreased to approx. 4.22 and 4.07 g/100g, respectively, compared with 4.73 g/100 g in the non-cultured milk. However, TS, protein and fat content showed only minor changes following culturing. Vitamin B content for both cultured products showed relatively minor changes, except for folic acid in zabadi which increased. Culturing led to increase in content and net utilization of calcium for both cultured milk porducts, especially acidophilus milk. The energy value in both cultured milk products were reduced. The energy value in both cultured milk products were reduced. The in vitro protein digestibility of zabadi and acidophilus milk was higher than of non-cultured milk, and the protein digestibility value obtained for zabadi was lower than the value obtained for acidophilus milk.

Akin and Konar (1993) investigated the effect of types of milk (cow or goat milk), flavourings (coffee, straberry, cherry or peach) and the duration of storage on the physio-chemical and organoleptic properties of yoghurt and indicated that the types of milk and flavouring had significant effect ($P < 0.05$) on the pH, titrable acidity, penetrometer readings and viscosity, but not on synersis. The colour and appearance, texture and taste and smell were affected ($P < 0.05$) by the type of milk and flavour, but not by duration of storage period. Yoghurt made from cow milk received higher ratings than that made from goat milk. The straberry yoghurts were rated the best followed by the peach, cherry and coffee varieties. This order of preference was not affected by the duration of storage.

Muir et. al. (1993) produced yoghurt with different levels of fat (0-10%) and sucrose (0-4%) and found that both fat and sucorse contents affected the sensory properties of yoghurt. Increasing fat content in milk improved creamy flavour and preceived viscosity key determinant of overall product acceptability in yoghurt. They also suggested that an optimum level for sugar addition is 1.2%.

Park (1994) evaluated the composition of eight varieties of commerical goat milk yoghurt (2 plain and 6 flavoured) produced in the USA and reported the mean percentage of TS, protein, fat, CHO and ash for plain yoghurt from three companies were $11.5 \pm 0.56, 3.99 \pm 0.12, 2.25 \pm 0.13, 4.49 \pm 0.56$ and 0.818 ± 0.019 respectively. Mean concentration (ppm on wet basis) for the pooled data of plain yoghurts were 1405 Ca, 149 Mg, 1253 P, 01417 K, 736 Na, 240S, 1.02 Fe, 0.345 Mn, 0.303 Cu, 3.37 Zn, 3.54 Al and 0.148 Mo. Plain varieties contained significantly ($P < 0.05$) lower TS and carbohydrate but significantly ($P < 0.05$) more protein and fat than the fruit varieties. Cherry-almond flavoured yoghurt had significantly ($P < 0.05$) lower ash than other varieties. Differences in Ca, Mg, Zn, P and Al levels between varieties for pooled or separate manufacturer data were significant (P < 0.05), whereas, K, Na and S were different only for separate manufacturer data. Correlation coefficient between levels of nutrients were variable with TS being significantly correlated with several nutrients, while Na, Mn and Mo did not correlate with any other parameters. The commercial goat milk yoghurt indicated that less dried skim milk and fruit were added to goat milk yoghurt.

Venkateshaiah et al. (1994) prepared yoghurt from cow whole milk (control milk) and a 50 : 50 blend of ground nut protein isolate (GPI) and cow whole milk (modified milk) by subjecting it to the following heat treatments (i) 85^0 C/30min, (ii) 90^0 C/30 min, (iii) steaming for 20 min. and boiling for 20 min. They found acid development in control and modified milk respectively, when incubated with yoghurt starter at 420 C/3.5 hrs after the various heat treatments, was (i) 0.75 and 0.66%, (ii) 0.76 and 0.68%, (iii) 0.70 and 0.64% and (iv) 0.76 and 0.62% lactic acid. Good quality yoghurt could be prepared from 50:50 cow milk : GPI blend that has been heat treated at 90^0 C/30 min.

Muir et. al. (1997) studied the relationship between composition and key sensory properties (creamy flavour, viscosity, and preceived serum separation) by preparing plain set yoghurt from pooled milk of Friesian cow of K-casein phenotype AA and that the sensory properties were related to TS content by K- casein phenotype had weak influence on serum separation only. Serum linkage diminished with increase in TS and was lowered in yoghurt made from K-casein AA than corresponding BB milk, greatest differences between phenotype being observed at the lower TS level.

Sensorial properties of ewe milk yoghurt had the highest qaulity followed by cow and goat milk (Pazakova et al. , 1999).

Plain and flavoured yoghurt made from goat milk culturing for 3 h 55 min at 40^0 C formed a slightly softer coagulum than that made from cow milk. Compared cow milk yoghurt, corresponding goat milk yoghurt, was slightly more acidic and less viscous and had slightly lower total sensory scores after 1, 3 and 9 days of storage. Highest sensory scores were noted after 3 days, when acceptability and desirability on hedonic scales, for plain peach and pistachio flavoured yoghurt respectively was 98.18, 96.96 and 100.0% for that made from cow milk and 80.0, 87.27, and 94.55% for that made from goat milk.

Real Del Sol et al. (2000) made yoghurt from a mixture of buffalo and cow milk flavoured with strawberry jam and studied the types of starter and the percentage of jam required by sensory and rheological evaluation. The results obtained indicated that the optimim starter was a 1: 1 mixture of the thermophilic cultures RR and B3 with 15% strawberry jam for flavouring.

Yeganehzad et. al. (2007) submitted that skim milk with 8.5% total solids was concentrated to 15 and 20% total solids by vacuum evaporation and inoculated with probiotic *Lactobacillus*. Yoghurts were incubated at 42 degress C and stored at 4 degrees C. Survival of *Lactobacillus*, physiochemical (pH, acidity, synersis, and hardness) and sensory properties (taste and texture) of probiotic yoghurts were evaluated every 7 day to 21 days. Results showed that, increasing the total solid concentration of milk increased the survival of *Lactobacillus acidophilus* the total solid concentration of milk increased the survival of *Lactobacillus acidophilus*, acidity and hardness of yoghurt and reduced the pH and synersis. However, the survival of probiotic *Lactobacillus* decreased throughout the storage period at 4 degrees C. This work shows the importance of total solic concentration of milk on survival probiotic strains, physiochemical and sensory properties of yoghurt.

Ghadge et. al. (2008) prepared buffalo milk yoghurts with the fortification of various proportion of either apple fruit pulp or honey, by the using mixed starter culture containing 1 : 1 ratio of Streptococcus thermophilus and Lactobacillus bulgaricus. The samples of fortified yoghurt were studied to determine the effects of fortification of apple fruit pulp and honey separately. The physical properties studied were setting time, syneresis, viscosity, while chemical properties were moisture content, acidity, pH and ash content. Sensory properties were evaluated by 9 point hedonic scale with the consumer taste panels to compare the properties of apple fruit pulp or honey fortified yoghurt with that of the control sample. The sensory properties evaluated were color, flavor, consistency, and overall acceptability. It is observed that yoghurts with superior sensory quality were obtained with 10% apple fruit pulp and 5% honey concentration.

2.2 Effect of Fat and SNF on Physico-chemical Quality of Yoghurt

Jennes and patton (1959) reported that the levels of total solids effect the titrable acidity of yoghurt mix due to buffering action of the protein, phosphate, citrate, lactates and other miscellaneous milk constituents.

Cottenie (1978) noted that thte evaporation of milk causes a change in calcium phosphorus caseinate system and this is beneficial for building up an optimum middle structure of protein which reduces or eliminate the tendency of wheying off.

On increase in total solid contents, increase the firmness of coagulum and enhance the rheological properties of yoghurt (Rasic and Kurman, 1978). The total solids level in milk for yoghurt manufactures can very from as low as 9.0% in skim milk yoghurt to over 20% in other type of yoghurt.

Humphreys and Plunkett (1969) reported that the increase in total solids, results in an increase titrable acidity and reduction in the coagulation time. The levels of milk powder addition varies from as little as 1% to as much as 6% (Stocklin, 1969). Generally recommended levels of fortification is around 3-4% (Becker, 1971). Robinson and Tamine (1975) recommended the TS level in the range of 14-18%.

Kozhev et al. (1970) produced bulgarian sour milk from cow milk which has been pastuirized at 92-95° C without or with holding (5, 10, or 15-20 min), increased TS level upto 18%, 7 levels (0.5-5%) of starter culture (*S. thermophilus* + *L.*

bulgaricus). They concluded that the best yoghurt was obtained from milk containing 15.5-16% TS, pastuirized at 92-95° C for 10 min, homogenized and incubated at 42° C and the amount. of starter culture added had no effect on the product quality.

Dordevic et al. (1973) suggested that total solids as high as 30.00 per cent. Tamine et al. (1987) showed that the chemical composition (percentage) of yoghurt (natural set and or/stired yoghurt) varied in total solids (12.0-18.7), fat (0.6-1.5), protein (4.5-6.4), lactose and other sugar (6.2-10.0), and ash (1.0-1.4). Tamine and Robinson (1988) showed that basic mix of yoghurt in concentrated to around 14-15 per cent solids. The level of solids also affect the titrable acidity of the mix due to the buffering action of protein, phosphates, citrates, lactates and other miscellaneous milk constituents.

Robinson (1977) prepared concentrated yoghurt from full cream spray dried milk reconstituted to 12-20% TS, incubating for 3.5 h with 2% starter culture and draining of whey from curd by placing in a cheese cloth bag. He found that an initial milk, TS content of 16% gave the most acceptable and product with a TS content of 23.44%, which was achieved by drainage of the yoghurt for 14 h in a refrigerator. Concentrated yoghurt containing < 20% TS was assessed as thin and tasteless, and that with > 25% TS become gummy and bitter.

Magdesi (1979) studied the effect of an addition of dried whole milk to liquid cow's milk on consistency and sensory properties of yoghurt coagulated at 42° C or 36° C. He prepared six sample consisting of liquid milk only; liquid milk with reconstituted milk in ratios of 5 : 5, 4 : 6, 3 : 7 and 2 : 8, and reconstituted milk only, fermented with 2% starter of *Streptococcus thermophilus + Lactobacillus bulbaricus*. The samples fermented at 36° C coagulated 1 hour latter than the samples fermented at 42° C. Finally, he reported that the reconstituted milk added in the different proportions had no effect on duration of the fermentation process and sensory properties of the final product unless used at levels > 70%. The fermented milks produced from mixtures of liquid and reconstituted milk, fermented at 36^0 C had better sensory properties than those coagulated at 42^0 C.

Richter et al. (1979) prepared yoghurt containing 0-4% fat, 0-6% sugar and 9-15% milk SNF and evaluated organoleptically by 50 peoples. They reported that the SNF was the most important component affecting the flavours, rheological and overall acceptibility of the yoghurt. Milk fat concentration was equally important in rheological acceptability. Sugar concentration influenced flavour acceptability more than over all or rheological acceptability.

Stoyanov and Radulov 91979) made yoghurt by the customary procedure using a L. bulgaricus / S. thermophilus (1: 2) starter from milk containing 3.6% fat alone or with addition of 1, 2 or 3% spray dried skim milk concentrate partly demineralized and delactosed by ultrafilteration and determined chemical composition, colour, aroma, taste, consistency, titrable acidity, pH, viscosity, synersis 30-120 min and microscopic structure of different yoghurt varients. After analysis of the data, they concluded that yoghurt made from milk supplemented with dried ultrafilteration concentrate had a firm coagulum, did not separate whey, had good aroma and pleasant taste and was organoleptically and rheologically superior to yoghurt made from milk with > 2% dried skim milk added, had a salty sweetish taste, whereas addition of 3% dried ultrafilteration concentrate had no such effect. The dry mater, protein, fat and lactose contents of the 3% dried ultrafilteration concentrate yoghurt were 15.13, 5.28, 3.46 and 4.29% respectively, vs 15.00, 5.09, 3.40 and 4.60% for 3% dried skim milk yoghurt.

Hong and Goh (1979) prepared yoghurt from milk corrected to 2-4% fat, heated for 30 min at 75, 85 or 90^0 C and incubated in the presence of a freeze dried starter culture for 2-3 h at 40 or 45^0 C. They found that titrable acidity immediately after 2 and 3 h incubation respectively were 0.53- 0.53 and 0.75 - 0.78% (as lactic acid) and after a further 24h at 5^0 C were 0.71- 0.74 and 0.90 - 0.93% respectively, the amount of acidity was not

significantly affected by differences in heat treatment at 95 or
75° C and it received the highest for yoghurt with 4% fat. The
ratio of streptococci : lactobacilli in 3 h culture was 5 : 5 at 40°
C and 2: 3 at 45° C and was 2 : 1, 1 : 1 and 2 : 3 after incubation
for 2, 3 and 4 h respectively at 42° C irrespective of fat.

Dolezalek and Vokacova (1981) studied the effect of several
factors on yoghurt quality, in several series of experiments. In
the temperature range of studied (70-90° C) heating milk to
80-90°C with 10 min holding was optimum giving yoghurt of
improved flavour and firm consistency. Of three incubation
temperature (30, 37 and 42°C) 42°C was the most effective
giving a product containing both starter organisms in about
equal compositions and having the best consistency, flavour and
aroma. Incubation size (0.2 for incubation at 30° C for 16 h, or
2% for incubation at 42° C for 3-4 h) affected lactic acid
fermentation and formation of acetaldehyde and free volatile
fatty acids, best final product being obtained with 2% inoculum
and incubation at 42° C. With increasing fat content of yoghurt
milk (from 0.05 to 3.5%), acidity contents of acetaldehyde and
free volatile fatty acids increased slightly and the quality of the
finished product improved.

Rasic and Kurman (1982) suggested that addition of about 2%
skim milk powder significantly improve the consistency of the
yoghurt. Addition of non fat dry milk is recommended to increase
the firmness of curd made from homogenized milk (Banks and
Evans, 1983).

Daraoui (1984) suggested the use of skim milk powder instead
of whole milk powder, because fat creates problem on the
manufacturing level for there is a risk of quality deterioration
arising from oxidation and development of nonacidity during
storage.

Lalas and Mantes (1985) collected 30 samples of strained
yoghurt, 30 of set type yoghurt and 20 of traditional Greek
yoghurt, each from 2 factories and taken retail outlets. In the
three types of yoghurt, the pH was 3.9 - 4.7, 3.9 - 4.4 and 4.0 -

4.2 with average values of 4. 32, 4.09 and 4.12 respectively. About 50% of strained samples contained lactic acid bacteria at only 10-1000/g, with the rest containing upto 10 million/g whereas about 90% of samples of the two others contained 10-95 million/g. Counts of other (contaminating) bacteria ranged from 10 to 680,000/g in all types of yoghurt, the traditional yoghurt having most samples with > 10000/g (60%). In virtually all of the stained and set samples, yeast count was < 25/g, whereas 50% of traditional samples contained 100-74000/g. The samples of strained and set yoghurt were of satisfactory microbiological quality, although the counts of starter bacteria in strained yoghurt were lower than the 100 million/g recommended by the FAO/WHO draft standard for live yoghurt. By contrast, the counts of contaminating bacteria, yeast and moulds in traditional yoghurt made in factories where too high.

Robinson and Tamime (1986) reported that in yoghurt milk proteins are responsible for the consistency and mounthfeel that distinguish it from other cultured milks, they also improved its nutritive value. Protein contents of milk to be processed into yoghurt is standaridized to 5%.

Shukla et. al. (1986) studied the effect of different stabilizers (gelatin, pectin, gum accacia, sodium alginate, sodium hexametaphosphate or carboxymethyl cellulose) on the diacetyl and volatile fatty acids contents of yoghurt made from milk standardized to 4.5, 3.0 or 1.5% fat. They recorded that the all stabilizers decreased diacetyl and volatile fatty acids (VFA) production as fat percentage in yoghurt decreased. Diacetyl and VFA production also decreased as compared to control without stabilizers.

Tamime et. al. (1987) examined the seven pots, each of flavoured and unflavoured fresh yoghurt and 2 x 2 pots of yoghurt stored at 5 or 10^0 C until the expiry date i.e. 12 - 14 days latter for chemical, bacteriological and sensory properties (appearance, colour, body and texture and flavour). They found that the fresh yoghurt was of good quality but stored at 10^0 C caused significant deterioration in quality. Protein, fat and sugars content in the yoghurts varied significantly (P < 0.001) in relation to source and flavour. Yoghurt pH could be correlated with manufature source. All coliform counts in this survey (fresh and stored yoghurt) testes were < 10 cfu/g, reflecting good sanitory manufacturing conditions. El-Deeb and Hassan (1987) examine the zabadi (yoghurt) chemically, microbiologically and organoleptically before and after storage at 5^0 C for 3, 5 and 7 days, made from standardized baffalo milk (4% fat) or lactose hydrolysed buffalo milk supplemented with defatted soyabean flour to 10,20 and 30 or 40% milk SNF. They concluded that quality of product made from lactose hydrolysed milk containing upto 30% milk SNF as soyabean flour was acceptable. Cold storage for upto 7 days caused decrease in sensory and pH values of zabadi and slight decrease in fat, total N and soluble tryptophane. Ratio of soluble N to total N, soluble tyrosine, volatile fatty acids, glucose + galactose, acetaldehyde and counts of lactic acid bacteria all increased during storage.

Garg (1988) reported that average composition of dahi made from whole milk was 85-88% water, 5-8% fat, 3.2-3.4% protein, 4.6-5.2% lactose, 0.70-0.75% ash, 0.5-1.10% lactic acid, 0.12-0.14% calcium and 0.09 to 0.11% phosphorus. Similar to this product yoghurt contained 17-25% DM and 83-75% whey (Chazinikolam, 1985).

Hofi (1988) made laben by pasturizing milk (8.7% TS), ultrafiltering at 50^0 C to 19% TS, standaridized retenate to 10% fat by adding 36% fat cream, inoculating with 3% yoghurt culture , filing and incubating at 42^0 C for 3.5 h, adding 0.5 NaCl then colling to 4^0 C. He found that the composition of this ultrafiltered (UF) and control (made from unconcentrated milk by traditional methods) respectively was TS 26.2 and 26.1, fat 9.8 and 10.0% protein 11.0 and 10.3%, lactose 3.96 and 3.56%, salt 0.45 and 0.53% and ash 1.52 and 1.14%. Organoleptic properties of the 2 labens were similar (appearance, body and texture, flavour). The UF methods gave higher yield of laben and shorter production time. Becker and Puhan (1989) studied the effect of increasing the SNF levels of milk to 9.0, 9.6 and 10.3% by addition of dried skim milk (DSM), by evoporation (EV) and by ulterafilteration on the rheological properties of yoghurt and indicated that viscosity of stirred yoghurt and firmness of set type yoghurt positively correlated with SNF content of milk. UF yoghurt had the highest viscosity and firmness in all cases. During storage for 2 week, UF yoghurt showed a lower post-acidification maximum (0.09 pH unit) than DSM and EV yoghurt (0.22 pH unit). No differences in sensory quality were observed between the different methods. The amount of milk needed for the manufacture of UF yoghurt increased than other methods, by 2.4% for 9.0% SNF, 4.3% for 9.6% SNF and 10.2% for 10.3% SNF.

Driessen et al. (1989) reported that a satisfactory viscosity was achieved for stirred yoghurts and other cultured products and creams without the used of additives of significant slime production by starter micro-organisms, addition of extra dried skim milk was only necessary in milk of < 4.0% fat. The viscosity of yoghurt reduced (stirred by shearing), but increased again after packaging and holding at < 10^0 C.

Cho-Ah-Ying et al. (1990) investigated the effect of incubation temperature (38 - 43°C) on the physio-chemical and sensory qualities of set and stirred yoghurt.The inoculum (3%) consisted of two types of yoghurt cultures, RR and SW in a ratio of 20 : 80 respectively. The two cultures contianed *L. bulgaricus* and *S. thermophilus* in a 1:1 ratio. The *S. thermophilus* strain in the RR culture produced polysaccharides. The results indicates that, there was no significant interaction between incubation temperature and type of yoghurt for titrable acidity, pH and viscosity, with respect to sensory qualities, the effect of incubation temperature was only significant for texture, viscosity, acidity, flavour and degree of liking were not affected.

Rathi et al. (1990) studied the physico-chemical properties of freeze dried dahi prepared by pre-freezing of dahi at -20^0 C, dyring for 12 h under a vacuum that decreased from 0.4 torr initially to 0.1 torr, to yield dried powder to 3.2% mixture that was filled into high density polythylene bags in a dry atmosphere, heat-sealed and stored in a desicator when at 40° C, it received of 6.67, 6.82, 6.77 and 6.45 vs 8.29, 7.29 and 7.72 for fresh dahi and overall acceptability scores was 6.45 vs 7.98. Physicochemical qualities of reconstituted and fresh dahi were as follow moisture 79.44 and 83.84%, TS 20.86 and 16.16%, pH 4.37 and 4.69, acidity 0.92 and 0.77%, diacetyl 8.13 and 11.13 mg/50 ml, curd tension 4.59 and 36.13g, and viscosity 150 and 919 cp at 30 rev/min. They also expressed his view that the lower curd tension and viscosity of the reconstituted dahi was due to complete destruction of the gel structure during the drying process.

Hassan and Mistry (1991) prepared low fat yoghurt by adding a newly developed dried milk (approx. 5% moisture, 84% protein, 2.0% fat, 0.7% lactose and 7% ash) to skim milk to obtain 5.1-10.9% total protein, 10.4-14.0% TS and < 0.1-4.5% lactose and mixtures were homogenized, pasteurized (90° C/10 min) and culture with a yoghurt culture at 45° C to pH 4.6. Thus, made yoghurt was compared with control yoghurt made from skim milk fortified with dried skim milk to 12% TS and concluded that yoghurt made with mixtures containing upto 5.6% protein, 10.5% TS and 3.75% lactose were similar in firmness, sensory scores when fresh and at 2 week, acetaldehyde content and fat content (< 0.2%) yoghurt with > 5.6% protein were firm and had an astrigent flavour.

Jogdand et al. (1991) made dahi by adding 0.1, 0.2 and 0.3% gelatin or sodium alginate to cow milk (4% fat), heating to boiling point and immediately cooling to ambient temperature then culturing at 42° C for 10 h with 2% streptococcus thermophilus/ Lactobacillus acidophilus (1 : 1) starter and reported that curd tension and viscosity increased while total volatile acidity and titrable acidity decreased with increasing level of either gelatin or sodium alginate. Sodium alginate in all cases having a greater effect than the irresponding level of gelatin. Overall acceptability of dahi was not significantly affected by either of the additives, and good quality was obtained using 0.1% sodium alginate.

Jogdand et al. (1991) prepared dahi from fresh cow milk supplemented with starch (0.5, 1.0 and 1.5%), sodium alginate (0.1, 0.2 and 0.3%) and gelatin (0.1, 0.2 and 0.3%), cultured with 1: 1 streptococcus thermophilus : Lactobacillus acidophilus starter and studied the effect of these additives on the quality of dahi. In this investigation they found that curd tension and viscosity increased while total acidity and total volatile acidity decreased with increasing levels of additives. sodium alginate had greatest and starch the least effect in all cases. Organoleptic studies showed scores of similar magnitude of all 3 levels of gelatin or sodium alginate, while dahi made with 1.5% starch had unacceptable consistency. Addition of 0.1% sodium alginate or gelatin or 1% starch is therfore, suggested for overcoming the wheying off problem and improving the quality of dahi.

Abd-Rabo et al. (1992) reported that soluble nitrogen and non-protein nitrogen gradually increased during incubation of goat milk yoghurt, whilst case in nitrogen and the mean lactose content decreased. Al-Saleh and Hammad (1992) investigated the quality of yoghurt prepared with the substitution of camel milk, camel milk butter, butter oil, cow milk butter, maize oil and sunflower oil at levels of 50, 75 and 100 per cent. Sensory evaluation indicated that yoghurt containing vegetable oil (maize and sunflower) was characterized inferior quality, whereas cow milk, butter oil, camel milk and camel milk butter produced good quality organoleptic properties of different yoghurt treatments. They recorded highly significant correlation between flavour and body of texture, flavour and total score, body and texture and total score as well as total score and overall quality.

Farooq and Haque (1992) showed the influence of sugar ester (0.05%) of various hydrophilic and lipophilic balances and textural properties of yoghurt. For this, fat free low energy yoghurt was assessed over 14 days storage at 4° C. Aspartame was used (200 ppm) to sweeten the skim milk based yoghurt that was established with starch (0.5%). The total solid content was 12.68% by weight. Sugar ester improve the over all quality of the yoghurt. Yoghurt with sugar esters mainly the stearates with hydrophilic-lipophilic balance range of 5 to 9, had better body, texture and mouthful than yoghurt without sugar esters, which were rated as coarse and grainy. The fat free low energy yoghurt sweetened with aspartame had fewer calories 101.4 (i.e. 50%) per 226.8 g (8-02) serving than regular yoghut containing 3.25% fat and 4% sucrose.

Sharma et al. (1992) reported that a increase milk solids in yoghurt from 14.7 to 20.4%, which was obtained by adding dried skim milk (2.8% w/v) to whole milk, increased the yield of freeze dried yoghurt from 0.2196 to 0.3067 $kg/m^2/h$. A reduction of 25.8% in drying time/unit output occured when the concentration of milk solids in yoghurt increased from 14.7 to 18.8%. A further increase in solid concentration, the yoghurt from 18.8% enhanced acceptability of product whereas a further increase in the level of milk solids imparted a chalky taste.

Chawala and Balachandran (1993) reported that yoghurt made from buffalo milk adjusted to 0.05, 1.5, 3.0, 4.5 and 6.0% fat respectively had mean rheological properties and sensory properties (scores) as follows : curd tension, 54.0, 29.0, 31.0, 37.0 and 42.0 g, penetration value 26.8, 26.0, 25.2, 24.4 and 23.0 mm, viscosity 25.0, 68.0, 145.0, 242.0 and 285.0 s/100 rev., before stirring and 28.0, 16.0, 27.0, 48.0 and 71.0 s/100 rev. after stirring. Sensory score (9-point hedonic scale) 4.98, 5.88, 7.14, 7.31 and 7.31 for flavour 5.62, 6.26, 7.12, 7.95 and 7.43 for body and texture and 6.52, 7.02, 7.14, 7.28 and 7.28 for appearance. Fat level had significant effect (< 0.01) on flavour, body and texture and apperance scores and results indicated that a levels of 3% fat in buffalo milk could be adequate for yoghurt manufacture.

Chawala and Balachandran (1994) investigated the effect of different levels (9.0 to 15.0%) of SNF in buffalo milk, revealed a higher culture activity at higher SNF levels with higher concentration of SNF in milk, curd tension and vistosity after stirring increased by 26.0 and 437.5 respectively and penetration value decreased by 5.9 per cent. Milk containing 3.0% fat and

10.0% SNF was found to be optimum for yoghurt preparation on the basis of sensory evaluation. When milk contained > 10.0% SNF sensory scores declined.,

Hofi et al. (1994) reported that satisfactory quality of zabadi was manufacture from milk fortified with dried skim milk (DSM), or ulterafiltered whey protein concentrate (UF-WPC) to 10-13% to increase the protein and TS content of zabadi and to reduce the whey disposal problem. The utilization of UF-WPC in the manufacture of zabadi yielded a product of higher nutritive value, firm coagulum, higher viscosity, reduced suceptibility to synersis compared with zabadi fortified with DSM. Organoleptically (for flavour and consistency) yoghurt fortified with DSM to 10% SNF and with UF-WPC to 10% SNF gave best results.

The two levels of fat and starter were added to the mixture of frozen yoghurt as follows : (a) 7% fat and 3% starter (b) 7% fat and 5% of starter (c) 10% fat and 3% starter and (d) 10% fat and 5% starter (Salem et al., 1994). Increasing fat content and starter inoculation during preparation of yoghurt, increase in titrable acidity and volatile. Acetaldehyde and organic acids (propionic, lactic, acidic and formic) increase until 15 to 60 days of storage. Increasing the viscosity of frozen yoghart mix resulted from increasing the viscosity of frozen yoghurt mix resulted from incorporating the starter culture and fat content. Viscosity had a clear effect on over-run which increased with the increasing fat content but decreases with increase in starter culture and fat content. Viscosity had a clear effect on over-run which increased with the increasing fat content but decreases with increase in starter culture concentration, after 9 days of storage. The coarseness of texture decreased with the increase in fat content but starter inoculum increases the coarseness slightly,.

Sakeel and Thompkinson (1994) studied the effect of different compositional and processing parameters on curd tension of filled bio yoghurt and reported the different levels of SNF and homogenization pressure had significant effect (P<0.01) on curd tension (CT). Fat levels also affected CT significantly (P < 0.05), while holding time at 90° C had no significant effect.

The product with higher fat (4.5%) and SNF (18.0%) levels homogenized 140.6/35.2 kg/m² and heated at 90° C for 30 min. had improved body texture characteristics with the highest CT value (39 gm).

Venkateshaiah et al. (1994) prepared yoghurt from milk standardized to 1, 2 and 3% fat, flavoured with 0.1, 0.2, 0.3 and 0.4% vanilla, pineapple or strawberry just before freezing in a soft-serve ice cream freezer. The investigation revealed that the flavour addition had little effect on over-run and melting resistance of the frozen yoghurt, but improved the acceptability of the product, optimum flavour levels were 0.4, 0.3 and 0.2 for vanilla, pineapple, strawberry respectively, and pineapple flavour was most acceptable. Falvour scores of all yoghurt increased with increase in fat levels. With scores (9-point hedonic scale) of 8.8, 8.3, 8.2 and 8.0 being recorded for pineapple , vanilla, strawberry and controlled yoghurt respectively made with 3% milk fat.

Vijaylakshmi et al. (1994) conducted a study on utilization of butter milk powder in preparation of low fat yoghurt. In manufacture of low fat yoghurt, dried butter milk was used to replace (i) 0.00 (ii) 25.00 (iii) 50.00 (iv) 75.00 (v) 100.00% of dried skim milk. Composition of (i) -(iii) respectively was fat 0.21, 0.50, 0.54, protein 4.88, 4.95, 4.91%, lactose 6.03, 6.08, 6.11% and T.S. 12.16, 12.21 and 12.23%. Corresponding values for acidity were 0.84, 0.85 and 0.80% lactic acid and for sensory scores (max. 20) were 0.84, 0.85 and 0.80% lactic acid and for sensory (max.20) were 18.98, 18.76 and 1883. It was concluded that replacement levels (ii) and (iii) produced low fat yoghurt with sensory, chemically and microbiological properties that were similar to control (i). Replacement level (iv) and (v) produced yoghurt of unacceptable quality.

Henny et al. (1995) showed that preparation of acidophilus milk from buffalo milk with 0.0 (skim milk), 1, 2, 3 percent fat by

heat treating at 90-95⁰ C/ minute and incubating at 37°C with
1 to 5% Lactobacillus acidophilus culture (Chg-Dri-Vac. culture)
until coagulation then stored at 7° C for 8 days. Titrable acidity
was directly related to size of inoculum and increased throughout
storage. L. acidophilus count reached a maximum on 4 days
then declined to levels lower than initial level. Total bacterial
count increased gradually throughout storage in samples with
1-2% inoculum but decreased again after 4 days in sample with
3-5% inoculum. Titrable acidity decreased slightly count
decreased at all storage periods. Total organoleptic scores were
the highest on days 2 to 4 of storage and acceptable acidophilus
milk could be prepared from 2% fat milk with 3% L. acidophilus
culture and stored for six days at 7° C.

McGlinchey (1996) conducted studies on the use of gelatin and
modified starches in yoghurt with reduced concentration of SNF
batches of yoghurt (fat content 1.5 or 3.5%) were prepared with
different concentration of milk SNF (12-14%), modified starch
(0.06%) and gelatin (0.03%). Rheological and sensory properties
of resulting yoghurt were also assessed. Both gelatin and
modified starch may be used in yoghurt without adverse effect
on quality. Modified starch with or without gelatin, was very
effective in low fat yoghurt. For yoghurt with higher fat content,
gelatin and modified starches gave the best result permitting
reduction of milk SNF concentration (and hence costs) without
impairing quality. It was concluded that modified starches permit
the manufacture of higher quality. It was concluded that
modified starches permit the manufacture of higher quality
yoghurt without added gelatin, and are hence suitable for
vegetarians.

Venkateshaiah et al. (1996) made yoghurt from milk adjusted
with cream to 3, 4, 5 and 6% fat and with dried SPM to 8.5,
10.5, 12.5 and 15.0% SNF and incubated with 3% starter to
acidity of 0.5, 0.5, 0.9 and 1.0% lactic acid, the yoghurt frozen
after addition of 18% sugar. Organoleptic analysis showed that
the optimum overall acceptability of frozen yoghurt was achieved
using milk containing 5% fat and 12.5% SNF and incubating

to 0.7% acidity. Higher levels of fat and SNF improved the body/texture but adversely affected flavour and overall acceptability.

Shaker et al. (2000) conducted a study on effect of fat content and preheat treatment of milk upon rheological behaviour of curd during the coagulation process of plain yoghur. Cream and skim milk were blended to given milk with 0.2, 0.8 and 1.5 and 3.0% fat and heated at 137^0 C/2s, homogenized at 13.79 Mpa, cooled at 40 C and packaged in 1 litre containers. To study the effect of milk preheat treatment, the standardized milk with 3% fat was heated at 137^0 C/2s, 90^0 C/3min, or 65 °C/30 min prior to homogenization, cooling and packaging. Viscosity of curd increased with fat content and was highest in milk pre heated at 137^0 C and lowest in that preheated at 65°C.

Kaminarides et al. (2007) reported charateristics of four type of yoghurt made from ovine milk containing 6.6%, 3.8%, 2.3%, or 0.9% fat, respectively. The yoghurt produced from ovine milk with high fat had the highest flavour and texture scores, fat and total solids content and firmness, but the lowest syneresis, lactic acid and galactose content. Low-fat yoghurts can be successfully produced from homogenised ovine milk and these yoghurts did not significantly differ from that of full fat yoghurt in values for ash, lactose, citric acid, pyruvic acid , pH and non-protein nitrogen. The HPLC procedure that was used for the determination of lactose was appropriate for the simultaneous determination of galactose and organic acids in milk or yoghurt . A total of sixteen volatile compounds were identified in ovine yoghurt and the main volatile flavour compounds in yoghurt on 2 days were acetic acid, acetaldehyde, acetone, diacetl, 2-butanone, 3-hydroxy-2-butanone and 3-methyl-2-butanone.

2.3 Effect of Starter Culture and Incubation Temperature on Physico-chemical Quality of Yoghurt

Galestoot et al. (1968), Moon and Reinbold (1978) and Shankar and Davis (1976) used the bacterial culture of *S*. thermophilus and *L. bulgaricus* in ratio of 1:1 to produce desired activity and characteristic flavour of yoghurt. The cocci bacilli ratio balances the more stable aroma production in yoghurt.

Higashio et al. (1978) identified growth factors for *S. thermophilus*, produced by *L. bulgaricus*, in milk which were valine, histidine, methionine, glutamic acid and leucine. A mixture of all five amino acids was required. Formic and pyruvic acids produced by *S. thermophilus* stimulated the growth of *L.bulgaricus*.

Madan Lal et al. (1978) examined three strains each of *S. thermophilus* and *L.bulgaricus* in various combinations for their symbiotic growth and production of good quality yoghurt. The combination of *S. thermophilus* (H) and *L. bulgaricus* (M) in the ratio of 1 : 2 and *S. themophilus* (H) and *L. bulgaricus* (M) in the ratio of 1 : 1 gave the best performance.

Singh and Kaul (1982) studied the activity of yoghurt starter in different types of milk. Cow's, buffalo's and goat's skim milks were heated at 100°C for 30 min, cooled to 37°C and inoculated with pure or mixed cultures of two strains of *S.thermophilus* (I and Hst) and *L. bulgaricus* (Yb, RTS and W). After incubation at 37°C for 24th, the acidity, acetaldehyde content and proteolytic activity of each culture was measured. Cultures grown in buffalo's milk produced more acidity and acetaldehyde and had higher proteolytic acivity than cultures grown in cow's and goat's milks. The yoghurt prepared from the three types of milk using three different mixed culture of *S. thermophilus* and *L.bulgaricus* strains, buffalo's milk yoghurt had the highest organoleptic scores.

Chawla and Balchandran (1985) found yoghurt culture (*S. thermophilus* and *L.bulgaricus*) in 1: 1 ratio at the rate of 3.0% to given the final product of desired sensory characteristics.

Kilic (1986) made yoghurt of good organoleptic quality from cow's milk by using liquid, frozen and freeze dried cultures of *S.thermophilus* and *L.bulgaricus* in the ratios of 1 : 1 and 0.8:1.2. The TS, lactose, acidity, acetaldehyde and yoghurt bacteria counts varied according to the cultures used. The highest yoghurt yoghurt bacteria counts were obtained with frozen cultures.

Nila et al. (1987) prepared fruit yoghurt by using 1 : 1 proportion of *S. thermorphilus* and *L. bulgaricus* in the rate of 3% inoculum. At the time of fermentation, differences in liberated amino acid was occured (Kapac et al., 1981) by using S. thermophilus and L.bulgaricus ratio 1 : 3 instead of 1 : 1 to obtain 1 : 1 ratio of *S.thermophilus* and *L.bulgaricus* in final product.

Kehagias et al. (1987) studied the fermentation of cow's, goat's and ewe's milk by thermophilic acid producing cultures. Milk from cow's, goat's and ewe's was incubated for 6 hours at 42-43° C with 3 yoghurt cultures-Wiesby V, Hansen CH-1, Rediset and Hansen B-3 Redi-set at 2.5% and then stored for 15 days at 4-7°C. The increase in acid and decrease in pH during culturing was greatest in ewe's milk and least in cow's milk, and was lower with Wiesby V than with the Hansen cultures. Proteolysis was also most marked in ewe's milk, which showed proteolysis throughout the culture period, whereas in goat's milk and cow's milk proteolysis reached a maximum and then decreased, especially with Hansen cultures. During storage, acidity of yoghurt increased from 0.8-0.9% for cow's and goat's milk and 1.0-1.1% for ewe's milk to 0.8-1.0% and 1.3-1.4%; final pH was about 4 in all cases. Overall, acetaldehyde tended to decrease with goat's milk and cow's milk and remain the same or size slightly with ewe's milk, acetaldehyde concentration tended to be highest with cow's milk. Proteolysis tended to continue during storage, with final free, tryosine concentration being 0.3 mg/g with cow's and goat's milk and 0.5 mg/g in ewe's milk. Penetrometer hardness, which was greatest for ewe's milk yoghurt, was not affected by storage, whereas, the viscosity cow's milk or goat's milk yoghurt, which was initially lower, remained same or tended to increase.

Gonc et al. (1988) reported that the yoghurt made from cow milk with 1.5 and 3.0% starter had better organoleptic properties when incubated at 42° C than when incubated at 48 or 54⁰ C. The amount of starter and the incubation temperature affected curd synersis but not stability or pH.

Robinson (1988) prepared three batches or natural yoghurt using the three starter culture, RR(^{N} 120), CH and B3 (Chr. Hansen's laboratory). Recorded the sensory attributes profiles (appearance, flavour, taste, mounthful and after taste) in the form of star diagram. He reported that yoghurt made with CH gave a strong profile with regard to flavour/acidity and curd irregularity. RR produced a smooth, slimy yoghurt, mild flavour and B3 had a good yoghurt flavour and a smooth viscous consistency. The optimum temperature for synergistic growth and metabolism, acid production, yoghurt viscosity and coagulum texture is 42°C.

Telles (1998) studied the biochemical activity of *S. thermophilus* and *L. bulgaricus* (1 : 1 ratios) during the manufacture and storage of goat milk and cow milk yoghurt. The manufacturing temperature was 43°C and samples were withdrawn at hourly intervals until the yoghurt become set. Storage temperature was 4°C and samples were withdrawn after 8, 16 and 24 h and 11 and 22 days. The studies included enumeration of the two organisms and determination of pH, titrable acidity, lactose content and free amino acid content, casein fraction content and proteolytic acvitivy. On the basis of result obtained it is concluded that the biochemical activity of the two organisms during yoghurt manufacture and storage was greater in goat milk than in cow milk.

Ghosh and Rajorhia (1990) studied the selection of starter culture for production of indigeneous Indian fermented milk product (Misti dahi). In this study 8 lactic acid starter cultures composed of (i) streptococcus lactic (C10), (ii) streptococcus thermophilus (HST), (v) *Lactobacilus bulgaricus* (LBW), (iv) a 1:1 mixture of C10 and DRC, (vii) a 1:1 mixture of HST and LBW and (viii) LF-40 a mixed culture of different stains of streptococcus lactis, streptococcus diacetylactis, streptococcus cremoris and leuconostoc, were tested for their ability to grow in a concentrated sweetened milk (18% milk solids and 14%

sucrose). On the basis of production of lactic acid, diacetyl and acetyl methly carbinol, pH and get firmeness obtained, the LF-40 culture was found to be the most suitable for commercial production of misti dahi.

Mehanna and Hefnawy (1990) conducted a study to evaluate the chemical changes during processing and storage of zabadi. In this study, zabadi was prepated by heating cow milk $+$ 2% dried SMP at 90°C/15 min, cooling to 45°C and inoculating with 2% yoghurt starter (1:1 *Streptococcus thermophilus/* Lactobacillus bulgaricus), incubating in plastic bottles at (42°C) C for four hour and storing at 6° C for upto 10 days. They found that the lactose content decreased from 5.68% initially to 4.68% and 3.68% during incubation and storage, respectively, and titrable acidity correspondingly increased from 0.25% initially to 0.80 and 1.24 per cent. Non protein N/OM increased slightly from 0.39 to 0.41% during incubation, than from 0.43 to 0.48% during storage, whilst acetaldehyde, present in trace amounts initially, increased to 22.0 ppm during incubation and to a peak of 68.00 ppm after storage for 6 days.

Hong et al. (1995) studied the effect of mixed strain culture on the texture and flavour of frozen yoghurt. They prepared frozen yoghurt using following freeze dried mixed cultures. ABT-containing *Lactobacillus acidophilus, Bifidobacterium langum* and *Streptococcus thermophilus*, ABY-2 containing *L. acidophilus, B. longum, S.thermophilus* and *L.bulgaricus* and YC-180 containing *L.bulgaricus* and *S.thermophilus*. Results showed that the frozen yoghurt made with ABT or ABY-2 had higher than that made with YC-180, and that made with ABT had the highedt scores for hardness, cohesiveness and elasticity. Sensory scores did not differ significantly between frozen yoghurt made with three cultures.

Aslim (1998) studied the metabolic products and antagonistic effect of combined *Lactobacillus bulgaricus* and *Streptococcus thermophilus* culture. He isolated and identified seven strains of *S. thermophilus* and seven strains of *L. bulgaricus* from yoghurt samples collected from different towns and villages of Turkey. These two strains were inoculated in proportion of 1:1, 1:2, and 2:2. Metabolic products and antagonistic effects were determined. The quality of metabolic compound produced by combined cultues was higher than that produced by single strains.

Skokanova et al. (1998) investigated the effect of culturing conditions upon final texture of stored yoghurt. For this, factors considered were : inoculum, which contained 50% *L.bulgaricus* and 50% *S. thermophilus*, with latter consisting of a 25/25, 0/25 or 50/0 mixture of strongly acidifying (A) and a highly texturing (T) strain; incubation temperature, 39, 42 and 45° C, final pH 4.4 and 4.8 and storage time 1, 7, and 21 days at 4°C. Using an equation based on weight of product, flow time and flow coefficient to characterize the flow properties of yoghurt, the texture was shown to be affected by type of strain. With *S.thermophilus.* T strain produce more viscous yoghurt and decrease with increasing culturing temperature and increasing final pH while there was no overall significant effect of storage upon texture. The texture of low viscosity yoghurt made with *S.thermophilus* increased significantly with storage time especially between days 1 and 7 when incubated to final pH 4.8.

Anjum et al. (2009) studied the effects of using two different starter cultures i.e. locally isolated starter culture and commercially imported starter culture (a mixed culture of *Lactobacillus bulgaricus* and *Streptococcus thermophilus*) and storage period on the chemical and sensory characteristics of yoghurt. For this purpose, four treatments of both cultures in combination (1 : 1) with different dose levels (1.5, 2.0, 2.5 and 3%) were used for yoghurt preparation. All these treatments showed different results. The pH of the samples displayed a decreasing trend for both types of yoghurts, but the decrease was relatively low in yoghurt made from commercially imported starter culture. Results for the acidity of the samples from both cultures revealed that the treatments and storage period have highly significant effect on the acidity of the samples whereas the interactions of treatments and storage period have non-significant effect on acidity. The total solids and lactose contents decreased gradually during the storage in both types of yoghurts, and the mean values showed significant effects of the interaction of treatments and storage period. The fat contents displayed non-significant results for treatments, storage period and their interaction. The mean values for sensory characteristics of the yoghurts for their taste, flavour, texture and overall acceptability were similar in both types of yoghurts for all treatments.

2.4 Effect of yoghurt Feeding on Growth rate, Feed Efficiency and Blood Profile in Rats

Astrup (1997) reported a fall in the serum cholesterol levels to the extent of 40% within a few weeks through daily consumption of four litres yoghurt, whereas Payers et al. (1977) and Thompson et al. (1982) reported no significant change in the serum cholesterol level in groups of six volunteers who consumed diets containing a high levels of yoghurt (1 to 1.5 litres/day) or an identical amount of milk or any other dairy product. Mann (1978) supported the finding of Astrup (1977) that substances present in milk that inhibit the cholesterol sysnthesis and gets enhanced by fermentation to yoghurt which consequently is responsible to lower serum cholesterol levels in human beings.

Mark and Howard (1977) reported that hypocholesterolaemic factor in milk is lactose. In the study they found that cottage cheese containing no lactose achieved no reduction in serum cholesterol while lactose (100 g/day, equv. to 4 pints milk) produce a reduction ($P < 0.05$) of about 7 per cent. However, they suggested that lactose is not the sole factor responsible for the reduction.

Hargrove and Alford (1978) reported that yoghurt had significantly greater, and directly acidified milk a much lower growth rate than other cultured milk or a control milk. The growth response was not observed if the yoghurt was sterilized after incubation, but was present if cultures containing

Streptocussus thermophilus were fed. *Lactobacillus acidophilus* was the only starter culture that could become established in the intestinal flora of the rat.

Hargrove and Alford (1978) studied the effect of yoghurt and other fermented milks on growth rate and feed efficiently in rats. They fed yoghurt and 3 types of acidophilus milk, lactic butter milk, Bulgarian butter milk and directly acidified milk, to rats in 6 different trials and reported that yoghurt gave greater weight gains than uninoculated control and other fermented milks. Its feed efficiency ratio was greater than the control in low fat milk but not in full fat milk. Rat fed directly acidified milk grewless well than rats on regular milk diets. Although additional vitamins stimulated growth in both yoghurt and the control but the superiority of the yoghurt was maintained. None of the other fermented milk gave improved growth of feed efficiency.

Hargrove and Alford (1980) conducted a study on growth response of weanling rats to heated, aged, fractionated and chemically treated yoghurt. The following treatments was given to freshly prepared yoghurt. (i) heated at 60, 65 or 70°C/2 min, (ii) treated with 0.03% H_2O_2, (iii) stored at 4.4°C for upto 4 week, (iv) freeze dried or (v) ultrafiltered. Findings indicates that feeding of yoghurt given treatments (i) significantly reduced weight gains by 20-25% (P < 0.01) and feed efficiency, (ii) and (iii), reduced weight gains but not feed efficiency. Freeze-dried yoghurt product greater weight gain but not feed efficiency. Freeze dried yoghurt produced greater weight gain than freeze dried milk. Feeding retenate from yoghurt with the permeate from milk resulted in greater weight gains than when permeate from yoghurt was fed with retenate from milk, indicating that the growth stimulant in yoghurt is present in the high mol. wt. fraction.

Massey (1981) observed no change in serum cholesterol concentration in group of 31 females supplemented with 450 gm of low fat yoghurt daily for 4 wks. The result did not indicate any hypocholesterolaemic effect of yoghurt except in individuals where high lipid concentration was reported.

Speck (1981) reported an interesting finding suggesting that cultured milk products contains a factor that inhibit blood cholesterol synthesis which makes it possible for lactobacilli to reduce the incidence of colon cancer. Stahelin et al. (1981) worked elaborately with four groups of pig. The animals were fed on high fat control feed for two weeks. Remaining three groups received simultaneously skim milk, yoghurt or casein for five weeks. After a further three week control feeding these groups were fed on whey, fermented whey or lactose for 6 weeks. The observation showed that skim milk decreased total serum cholesterol and high density lipoprotein (HDL) cholesterol by 13-14%, respectively. Yoghurt had similar effect on HDL cholesterol but less on total cholesterol, casein had no significant effect. Whey and fermented whey decreased total cholesterol slightly but HDL cholesterol considerably (15%). These findings are duly supported by the observations of Thankur and Jha (1981) who worked with five groups of rabbit over a period of 16 weeks. The control group received the stock diet, the other four groups received cholesterol at 0.1 mg/kg body weight without or with 20ml milk, 20 ml yoghurt and 15 mg CaCO3. Mean serum cholesterol, the yoghurt and calcium were identical in this regard indicating marked reducing effect.

Mc Donough et al. (1982) assessed the growth in rats fed with freeze dried (FD), liquid milk and yoghurt. They found that wt. gains of rats on yoghurt were 24.3% higher than for milk when fed as liquid and 24.6% higher when fed freeze drid. Feed effeciency for yoghurt diets were significantly higher than for milk diets.

Bazzare et al. (1983) studied the effect of yoghurt and calcium supplementation on total cholesterol and HDL cholesterol of blood in womens and men and reported that mean total cholesterol decreased significantly in women after they had taken yoghurt and also decreased after they had taken calcium but not significantly. Mean high desnity lipoprotein (HDL) cholesterol and HDL cholesterol : total cholesterol ratio for women were greater after yoghurt and calcium supplementation. Total cholesterol : HDL cholesterol ratio for men not different at any time.

Hitchins et al. (1983) reported that stimulation of weanling rat growth by yoghurt and related fermented milk was associated with increased feed efficiency and increased consumption. During the 4 week bioassay the importance of stimulation depended inversely on growth performance of control rats. Stimulation was unrelated to final pH, lactose content or bacterial lactase content, but was related to bacterial content. Lactobacillus bulgaricus could be omitted from the yoghurt fermentation or replaced by the other bacteria without reducing stimulation. Lactase pretreatment of control milk improved growth performance.

Massey and Davidson (1983) studied the effect of lactose content of non fat milk diets on male rat serum lipids and lipoproteins. For this groups of rats were fed 1 to 3 different semisynthetic diets based on skim milk but containing decreasing amount of lactose from, respectively dried skim milk, yoghurt or lactose hydrolysed milk. A 4th groups received a standard laboratory diet. After feeding for 28 days energy consumption, growth rate, feed efficiency, liver cholesterol and triglyceride concn. were similar for the 4 groups. Although no hypocholesterolaemic effect of the milk based diets was observed, significant differences in serum lipoprotein pattern were found. β−lipoprotein content was lower with all 3 milk based diets than with the control diet, fast alpha-lipoprotein decreased while the slower alpha-lipoprotein increased as the lactose content of the diet decreased. Results indicate that lactose containing food may alter the risk of atherosclerosis even when total serum lipids and total high density lipoprotein concn. are unchanged.

Wong et al. (1983) studied the origin of growth stimulating factor in yoghurt, liquid or freeze-dried diets of milk, milk fermnented by Streptococcus thermophilus or Lactobacillus bulgaricus, and milks to which cells of S.thermophilus or L. bulgaricus were added by feeding it to rats. Diets containing sonicated cells, all supernatant, and cell fractions also were fed. The observations indicate that milk fermented by S.thermophilus and milk plus S. themophilus cells stimulated growth as effectively as did yoghurt. This finding and the absence of stimulation in rats fed L. bulgaricus showed that S. thermophilus is responsible for stimulation of growth by yoghurt. Growth was stimulated by a intracellular factor and not by fermentative changes in the milk.

Jaspers et al. (1984) fed 10 humen adults with usual diets modified by incorporating 681 g nonfat and unpasteurized yoghurt daily throughout 14-21 day periods. They reported that daily consumption of yoghurt significantly reduced fasting total serum cholesterol 10-12% in human adult male on some days, but serum cholesterol returned to control values with continued yoghurt consumption. Serum triglycerides and proportions of serum lipoproteins were not significantly influenced by increasing yoghurt consumption.

Ishida and Kubo (1985) examined the effect of yoghurt, kefir, and butter milk on serum lipids in rats and found that feeding of bifidus yoghurt (@ 15% to chow or control) to 10 weeks old female wistar rats for 28 days, decreased total cholestrol, HDL-cholesterol, triglyceride and phospholipid in serum but increased total cholesterol in liver (P < 0.01) in their first trial. In second trial they reported that feeding of heat treated kefir @ 15% of chow) + cholesterol (@ 1% of chow) and sodium deoxycholate (@ 0.3% of chow) with chow (control) for 14 day increased the total cholesterol and triglycerides but decreased HDL-cholesterol in total cholesterol in serum of 12 week old male rats compared with control. In their third trial, they reported that feeding or butter milk @ 7.5% of chow) for 10 days had no effect on cholesterol or lipid in serum of 9 week old female rats, but adding cholesterol @ 1% to chow or chow + butter milk decreased HDL cholesterol concentration by 50 per cent.

Wong et al. (1987) reported the feeding of Sprague- Dawley rats, initially weighing 45 to 55 g, with milk based diets, 50% yoghurt casein, 50% yoghurt whey or yoghurt. They found weight gains after 4 weeks 112.5, 145.3, 62.3 and 126.5g respectively. In another trial rats were given diets with yoghurt, 50 or 25% yoghurt casein, 50% reference casein, 50 or 25% cultured butter milk or milk. Yoghurt diets contained Sterptococcus thermophilus and Lactobacillus bulgaricus and butter milk diets contained S. lactis and S. cremoris. After 4 week feeding weight gains were 138.1, 189.0,150.0, 144.6, 153.4, 144.8 and 116.2 g.

Kaup (1988) reported that feeding of rats with fermented yoghurt and unfermented yoghurt with added lactic acid resulted in improved bone formation, whereas, high levels of dietary calcium resulted in increased bone Ca and improved bone formation and reduced the levels of serum cholesterol and serum triglycerides in blood. Rat fed yoghurts had lower serum cholesterol levels than rats fed $CaCO_3$ and rats fed unfermented yoghurts with added acid had lower serum cholesterol levels than rats fed unfermented yoghurt with no added acid. Lee et al. (1988) reported that rats fed diets containing either heated mix or yoghurt tended to eat more and gain more weight than that feds diets containing either unheated mix or the acidified yoghurt. Feeding efficiency was also significatly higher for rats fed heated mix and yoghurt.

Danielson et al. (1989) isolated three strains of Lactobacillus acidophilus (LA) from faeces of mature boars that were not being fed antibiotics from the Nebraska Gene Pool (NGP). All LA isolates were screened in vitro for anticholesterolaemic and antimicrobial activities. One strain, LA 16, caused the greatest reduction in cholesterol and inhibited Bacillus subtilis and Escherichia coli. LA 16 was used to produce Acidophilus yoghurt (AY). All he 18 boars were fed on a high cholesterol 6.661 g daily. Nine boars were given 1.81 kg daily of a second diet supplemented with AY 0.454 kg daily. The other nine boars were given the original diet. Cholesterol intake was the same for the 2 diets. AY reduced serum cholesterol and low density lipoprotein cholesterol but it had no effect on serum triglycerides or high density lipoproteins.

Mc Namara et al. (1989) studied the effect of yoghurt intake on plasma lipid and lipoprotein concentration in 18 normolipaemic men during 3 dietary phases. In phase I low fat, low cholesterol baseline diet was eaten for 3 weeks. The baseline diet supplemented with low fat yoghurt (16 oz daily) was eaten for 4 weeks during pharse II and during phase III the supplement consisted a non formented dairy product (16 oz low fat milk +10% milk solids). In their study they found that the average body weight and dietary intake of fat, cholesterol and polyunsaturate : saturate fat ratios were not significantly different for the 3 dietary phases. Plasma, total, LDL and HDL were not affected by the yoghurt or the low fat milk concetrate.

Navder et al. (1990) investigated the effect of skim milk, skim milk yoghurt, orotic acid and uric acid on lipid metabolism in rats. They fed Sprague Dawley rats with isoenergetic diets without or containing 45% SM, 45 SM yoghurt, 0.0025% orotic acid (OA) or 0.001% uric acid (UA), without or with 0.5% cholesterol and reported that SM + cholesterol decreased the total cholesterol ($P < 0.10$), low density lipoprotein (LDL) cholesterol ($P < 0.05$) aortal cholesterol ($P < 0.01$) and liever cholesterol ($P < 0.10$) and increased high density lipoprotein (HDL) cholesterol ($P < 0.05$) and HDL/LDL cholesterol ratio ($P < 0.01$) and increased LDL cholesterol ($P < 0.05$). The hypercholesterolaemic effects were greater for SM than for SMY. OA and UA increased serum cholesterol, LDL cholesterol and total liver lipids, the OA diet also increased liver cholesterol.

Goh et al. (1994) studied the effect of ginseng-yoghurt on the blood glucose, serum cholesterol and inhibition of cancer in mouse and reported that feeding of control diet containing 20% casein, modified control diet with 10% yoghurt (CY) or 10% ginseng (CG) or ginseng-supplemented yoghurt (CGY) had no significant effect on glucose levels in mice but mean levels at 3 weeks were lower in mice fed CG or CGY than in those fed CY or control diet (103.0 and 101.7 vs 112.7 and 111.3 mg/dl, resp.). Mean serum cholesterol level (in mg/dl) at 3 weeks in mice fed control, CY, CG and CGY diets, respectively, were as follows :

total cholesterol - 65.2, 71.2, 77.5 and 79.2 low density lipoprotein (LDL) cholesterol 93.4, 73.8, 58.8 and 62.3, free cholesterol 47.8, 43.2, 40.7 and 41.1 and cholesterol ester 110.8, 101.8, 95.6 and 100.4. In tumour induce ICR mice feeding of ginseng inhibit growth of ascities tumour cell althouth the inhibition was not significant but no inhibitory effect on solid form sacroma was observed.

Moussa et al. (1995) studied effect of fresh cow's milk and some fermented milk products on rat serum cholesterol, triglycerides, total lipids and lipoprotein. They used the following diets for the feeding of 30 mature albino rats, devided into 6 groups, for 30 days; (i) dry diet alone (control I) or together with (ii) fresh cow milk (control II), (iii) fresh yoghurt, (iv) biograde. At end of the feeding period blood sample was taken and analysed for total, high and low density lipoprotein cholesterol, triglycerides and total lipids and reported that with exception of HDL cholesterol, serum of rat receiving (ii) diet, whereas, feeding of any of cultured milks reduced the levels. The reduction in serum cholesterol, triglycerides, total lipids and LDC cholesterol varied between type of cultured milk but their overall benefits was placed in the order (v) > (vi) > (iv) > (iii).

Suzuki (1995) investigated the effect of cultured milk on serum lipid metabolism using 41 strains of lactic acid bacteria and reported that L. adidophilus LA 2050 was the most effective strains in preventing elevation of serum cholesterol concentration when administered as cultured milk to rats fed a high cholesterol diet.

Poppel and Schaafsma (1996) explained that consumption of yoghurt (cultuted with traditional yoghurt starter culture and two strains of L. acidophilus as probiostics), 3 x 125 ml daily in combination with breakfast, lunch and diner significantly decreased serum total cholesterol (by 4.4%), LDL-cholesterol (by 5.4%) and the LDL-HDL cholesterol ratio (by 5.3%) when compared with control.

Akalin et al. (1997) investigated the effect of yoghurt and acidophilus yoghurt on the live weight gain, serum cholesterol, HDL, and LDL-cholesterol, triglycerides and number of faecal lactobacilli and coliform in mice assigned to 3-dietary groups (n = 20/group) for 56 days, (i) commercial rodent chow + water (control), (ii) commercial rodent chow + yoghurt made from milk inoculated with a 3% (V/V) liquid culture of S. thermophilus + L. delbrueckii subsp. bulgaricus and (iii) commercial rodent chow + yoghurt made from milk inoculated with a 0.01% (W/V) freeze dried culture of S. thermophilus + L. acidophilus. The liveweight gain of (ii) and (iii) mice were higher than those of (i) mice. The mean values for serum cholesterol concentration and LDL-cholesterol concn. were significantly decreased when (iii) was fed on days 28 and 56. HDL-cholesterol and triglyceride were not affected by (ii) and (iii). The highest number of faecal lactobacilli and the lowest number of faecal coliforms were found in (iii) mice.

Beena and Prasad (1997) investigated the effect of yoghurt and bifidus yoghurt fortified with skim milk powder, condensed whey and lactose hydrolysed condensed whey on serum cholesterol and triacylglycerols levels in rats. They fed following diets to rat, (i) basal diet (control), (ii) basal diet + cholesterol, (iii) as (ii) + whole milk, (iv), (v) and (vi) as (ii) + standard yoghurt fortified with dried skim milk powder, condensed whey, or lactose hydrolysed condensed whey, respectively, and (vii, viii and ix) as (ii) + bifidus yoghurt containing Bifidobacterium bifidum + the 3 additives respectively, cholesterol was 5g/kg body weight. After 30 days, triacylglycerols, total cholesterol, high density lipoprotein (HDL) cholesterol and low density lipoprotein (LDL) cholesterol levels were measured in blood serum. Group (ii) and (iv) had no cholesterolaemic effect but (vi), (vii), (viii) and (ix) lowered serum cholesterol yoghurt increased the concentration of triacylglycerol in rat. This studies has shows that bifidus yoghurt and yoghurt fortified with whey protein can reduce total and LDL-cholesterol in rats.

Kar et al. (1998) evaluated the effect of the consumption of unpasteurized and pasteurized freshly prepared acidophilus yoghurts were fed to 2 groups of volunteers (n = 11 group, 45-55 years old) for 4 weeks (the unpasteurized yoghurt contained on average 7 x 108 cells/g, subjects received 200g/day). Serum cholesterol was determined before, after 2 and 4 weeks of the trial and 2 weeks after the end of the study. Both products showed a significant effect on serum cholesterol concentration. There was also significant variation on serum cholesterol among the volunteers. However, there was no significant differences between the effect of the unpasteurized and pasteurized yoghurt on serum cholesterol.

Anderson and Gilliland (1999) conducted a two controlled clinical studies to examine the effect of consumption of 1 daily serving of cultured milk (FM) (yoghurt) on serum lipids. In the first study, subjects were randomaly allocated to FM containing L. acidophilus L1 of humen origin or to FM containing L. acidophilus ATCC 43211 of swine origin. In this single-blind study, subjects consumed 200-ml serving of FM daily for 3 weeks. The second study was a double blind, placebo-controlled, cross over-study. Subjects completed a 4 week first treatment, had 2-week washout and completed a second 4- week treatment. In the second study, subjects consumed FM containing L. acidophilus L1 or placebo FM containing L. acidophilus L1 was accompanied by a 2.4% (P < 0.05) reduction of serum cholesterol concentration. In the second study, strain L1 reduced serum cholesterol concentration. In the second study, strain L1 reduced serum cholesterol concentration by 3.2% (P < 0.05) in the first treatment period. In the second treatment period there were no significant changes in serum cholesterol concentration. Combined analysis of the 2 L1 treatment studies demonstrated a 2.9% (P < 0.01) reduction in serum cholesterol concentration. It is concluded that because every 1% reduction in serum cholesterol concentration is associated with an estimated 2-3% reduction in risk for coronary heart disease, regular intake of FM containing an appropriate strains of L.

acidophilus has the potential of reducing risk for coronary heart disease by 6-10%. Roos et al. (1999) reported that yoghurt enriched with L.acidophilus L-1 does not lower serum cholesterol in men and women with normal to borber line high cholesterol levels.

Agerholm et al. (2000) fed 450 ml yoghurt daily to four groups of men and women during the study of effect pf probiotic milk products on risk factors for cardiovascular disease. Group 1 received yoghurt fermented with 2 stains of S. thermophilus and 2 strains of L. acidophilus (St La). Group 2 : fed with a plucebo yoghurt fermented with delta acid lactone. Group 3 : received a yoghurt fermented with 2 strains of S. thermophilus and one strain of L. rhamnous (St Lr.) Group 4 : received a yoghurt fermented with one strain of Enterococcus faecium and 2 strains of Streptococcus thermophilus. (CAUSIDO culture). The 5th group was given 2 placebo pills daily. After comparing all 5 treatment groups,, unjusted for changes in body weight, no statistical effects were observed in 8 week in the G-group on low density lipoprotein (LDL) cholesterol (P = 0.29). After adjustment for small changes in body weight LDL-cholesterol decreased by decreased by 8.4% (0.26 $\pm$ 0.10 m mol litre, P < 0.05) after 8 weeks in G-group. This was significantly different from the group consuming chemically fermented yoghurt and the group consumed placebo pills (P < 0.05). The CAUSIDO culture reduced LDL-cholesterol and increased fibrinogen in the overweight subjects at a 450 ml consumption daily.

Kedar et al. (2000) investigated the effect of maize oil or butter without bacterial strains and butter diets supplemented with yoghurt (Bifidobacterium bifidum and Lactobacillus acidophilus) strains and their mixture on the total serum cholesterol, HDL-cholesterol and LDL-cholesterol and triglycerides levels, as well as, saturated and unsaturated fatty acids and the total cholesterol of liver tissue in rats. They reported that supplementation of butter diets with yoghurt or probiotics strain significantly reduced the serum cholesterol, HDL and LDL-cholesterol and triglycerides levels while their mixture had the lowest amount of total choesterol, LDL and triglycerides levels. Bacterial strains had higher unsaturated fatty acids level than saturated fatty acids levels, but reduced cholesterol in rats liver tissue. Corn oil diets without bacterial stains increased faecal entreococci and faecal coliform, while they reduced faecal lactobacilli. Supplementation of butter diets with either yoghurt or probiotics strains reduced the number of both faecal enterococci and coliforms, but increased the number of both faecal enterococci and coliforms , but increased the number lactobacilli. L. acidophilus showed the highest capability to reduce the growth of both enterococci and coliforms followed by B. bifidum and yoghurt stains. Rats fed with B. bifidum diets exhibited higher number of lactobacilli in their faeces than rats fed with butter diets without these bacterial strain. The use of mixture of yoghurt and probiotic strains reduced the growth of enterococci and coliforms in the intestinal tract.

Al-Wabel et al. (2008) studied the biological effects of aqueous herbal extracts mixed with stirred yoghurt filtrate against alloxan-induced oxidative stress and diabetes in rats. Aqueous extracts of six medicinal plants : fenugreek, greater burdock, goat's rue, colocynth, chicory and lupine were mixed with stirred yoghurt filtrate and used in the experiments. Blood glucose and alanine and asparate amino transgerase (ALT and AST) activities were estimated before and after alloxan-induced oxidative stress and diabetes in rats. Obtained results showed that blood glucose levels in sera of treated rats fed on aqueous extract of medicinal plants and stirred yoghurt filtrate mixture decreased with mean values of 135.0 + or - 26.85 mg/100 ml serum compared with the treated rat fed on basal diet (positive control) with mean value of 237.66 + or -14.43 mg/100 ml serum. Data showed that ALT and AST activities in sera of treated rat fed on aqueous extract of medicinal plants and stirred yoghurt filtrate mixture were nearest to the level of un-treated rats fed basal diet (negative control). The means values of ALT and AST level in treated group fed on aqueous extract of medicinal plants and stirred yoghurt filtrate mixture were 57.33 + or -20 and

189.33 + or -48.85 compared with the positive control 90 + or -31.76 and 260.00 + or 57.27 and negative control 44.66 + or -9.5 and 180.66 + or -23.58 UL⁻¹, respectively. Data concluded that mixture of medicinal plant extracts and stirred yoghurt filtrate may play a role in protection against alloxan-induced oxidative stress and diabetes in rat.

Rossi et al. (2008) obtained an isoflavone-supplemented soy yoghurt, fermented with Enterococcus faecium CRL 183 and Lactobacillus helveticus ssp jugurti, with suitable sensory properties and to assess the effects of the final product on blood lipids in hypercholesterolemic rats. Four isoflavone supplementation procedures were tested, in which the isoflavone was added at these stages : (1) before heat-treatment; (2) after heating and before fermentation; (3) after fermentation and (4) in the okara (by-product of soy milk) flour stirred into the fermented product when consumed. The products were subjected to a test of sensory acceptability, To assess their potential hypocholesterolemic properties in vivo, four groups of rats were used : control (C), hypercholesterolemic (H), hypercholesterolemic plus fermented product (HF). Hypercholesterolemia was induced in rats of groups H, HF and HFI by feeding them on a commercial rat chow to which cholesterol and cholic acid had been added. Total, HDL and non-HDL cholesterol and triglycerides were measured in the blood of the rats. No significant sensorial differences were detected among the samples of soy yoghurt supplemented with isoflavones at various processing stages. Rats fed a fermented soy product enriched with isoflavones (HFI group) had significantly ($P > 0.05$) less serum total cholesterol (15.5%) compared with rats fed a hypercholesterolemic diet (H group). Non-HDL cholesterol was less ($P < 0.05$) in rats fed a fermented soy product enriched or not with isoflavones (27.4 and 23.2%) compared to H group. The HDL-C and triglyceride concentrations did not differ significantly among the groups. It was possible to obtain an isoflavone-supplemented soy yoghurt with satisfactory sensory characteristics. The resulting supplemented soy yoghurt was capable of producing a lipid-lowering effect in hypercholesterolemic rats, relative to the animals that did not consume this product.

Gowder and Halgowder (2008) fed food flavor cinnamaldehyde (CNMA) orally to the rats at the dose 2.14, 6.96, 22.62 and 73.5 mg/kg body weight/day for 10, 30 and 90 days. Only the group of rats treated with CNMA at the dose 73.5 mg/kg body weight/day for 90 days showed histological changes in the kidney followed by increased activities of renal, serum and urinary enzymes. CNMA-induced glucosuria in these rats was accompanied by marked proteinuria and creatinuria and creatinuria. Increased serum blood urea nitrogen and serum creatinine and decreased serum protein and glucose levels were observed in these rats. Thus, CNMA at the dose of 73.5 mg/kg body weight/day for 90 days exert its effect on kidney of male albino wistar rat and its effect is time and dose dependent group hypercholesterolaemia model group and experimental groups I and II according to serum total cholesterol (TC), triglyceride (TG), high density lipoprotein cholesterol (HDL-C) and low density lipoprotein cholesterol (LDL-C) concentrations. The control group was fed a basic diet while the 3other groups were fed a high-fat diet. The experimental groups were given the test substances intragastrically for 8 weeks, while the control and model groups were given water. The serum TC, TG, HDL-C and LDL-C concentrations were determined at the end of the 2nd, 4th, 6th and 8th weeks. Compared with the model group, the serum TC, TG and LDL-C levels were significantly decreased while the HDL-C level was increased after 8 weeks of treatment in the experimental group, with group I having better results than group II. It is concluded that CBL from kefir grain has significant cholesterol-reducing effects in hypercholesterolaemic rats.

Abdel- Salam et al. (2009) formulated a functional yoghurt cake using hot water extract of stevia leaves as a sweetener. The ingredients of the regular yoghurt cake were replaced by both low caloric value and functional ingredients. Sucrose was replaced by hot water extract of stevia, butter was replaced by egg white and 72% extraction wheat flour was replaced by whole flour.Orange peels and lemon rind were also added to the formulated yoghurt with stevia extract. Sensory evaluations for both the regular yoghurt cake and formulated yoghurt cakc for diabetics were carried out using scores of the appearance, colour odor, flavor, texture and overall acceptability. The obtained results showed that the regular yoghurt cake and formulated yoghurt cake for diabetics have a good score. The biological evaluation of rat blood parameters of control and yoghurt cake of diabetics evaluation of rat blood parameters of control and yoghurt cake for diabetics groups showed that bilirubin, high-density lipoprotein (HDL) cholesterol, triglycerides, cholesterol, creatinine, alkaline phosphatase, blood glucose and gamma-glutamyl tranpeptidase (gamma -GT_ values (means) in yoghurt cake for diabetics group were similar to results obtained in regular yoghurt cake group. There was a slight decrease in urea and aspartate aminotransaminase (AST) (37.05 mg/dl and 86.82 U/L, respectively) values in yoghurt cake for diabetics group compared with control (43.26 mg/dl and 97.00 U/L, respectively).

7 Yoghurt Technology and Experimentation

The present investigations was carried out in the Department of Animal Husbandry and Dairying, Institute of Agricultural Sciences, Banaras Hindu University, Varanasi (Kumar, 2002). The details of the materials used and the techniques followed during the course of investigation have been described hereunder :-

Phase I - Standardization of milk for yoghurt manufacture

3.1 Procurement of raw materials

3.1.1 Procurement of milk (Cow and Buffalo) - Fresh milk was collected daily in the morning from the bulk of cow and buffalow milk available at B.H.U. Dairy Farm daily.

3.1.2 Procurement of Cream - During the course of aforesaid investigations cream was separated daily in the laboratory by hand driven cream separator. The cream, when not used immediately, was stored in a refrigerator to avoid acid development. Invariably fresh cream was used after pasteurization.

3.1.3 Skim milk powder - Skim milk powder (AMUL- spray dried) having 97% TS (99% fat free) was bought from the open market and used in calculated amount for preparation of yoghurt.

3.1.4 Starter culture - Frozen dried strains of Streptococcus thermophilus and Lactobacillus bulgaricus were obtained from National Collection of Dairy Cultures (NCDC), Dairy Microbiology Division of NDRI, Karnal, Haryana. These strains were developed in the laboratory of Department of A.H. &

Dairying, B.H.U., Varanasi. The individual stain of microbes in desired ratios were used for manufacture of yoghurt.

3.1.5 Plastic containers and parchment paper - Plastic containers (100 gm capacity) and plain butter paper (wrapper) were bought from the open market of Varanasi.

3.2 Experimental Details

3.2.1 Desing of experiment

The investigation entitled "Technology and Nutritional Aspects of Yoghurt" designed as a Factorial Completely Randomized Block Design experiment involving three levels each of fat and SNF; two levels of temperature; five ratios of starter culture and two sources of milk viz., cow and buffalo milk. The treatments were replicated thrice as shown in Table 1.a and 1.b.

Table 1a : Symbolic presentation of different treatment combinations

Sources of milk (M)	Fat (%) (F)	SNF (%) (S)	Temp (^{0}C) (T)	Starter culture/ratio (ST)
Cow milk (M_1)	4 (F_1)	10 (S_1)	39 (T_1)	Set1 (SL 1:1)
	5 (F_2)	11 (S_2)	42 (T_2)	Set2 (SL 1:2)
	6 (F_3)	12 (S_3)		Set3 (SL 1:3)
				Set4(SL 2:1)
				Set 5 (SL 3:1)
Buffalo milk (M_2)	do	do	do	do

3.3 Preparation of yoghurt samples

3.3.1 Ingredients used

(i)   Fresh cow and buffalo milk

(ii) Fresh cream

(iii) Spary dried skim milk powder.

Table 1b : Permutation combinations of treatments (one hundred eighty treatment combinations)

Symbol	Treatment combination	Symbol	Treatment combination	Symbol	Treatment combination	Symbol	Treatment combination
T_1	$M_1T_1F_1S_1ST_1$	T_{46}	$M_1T_2F_1S_1ST_1$	T_{91}	$M_2T_1F_1S_1ST_1$	T_{136}	$M_2T_2F_1S_1ST_1$
T_2	$M_1T_1F_1S_1ST_2$	T_{47}	$M_1T_2F_1S_1ST_2$	T_{92}	$M_2T_1F_1S_1ST_2$	T_{137}	$M_2T_2F_1S_1ST_2$
T_3	$M_1T_1F_1S_1ST_3$	T_{48}	$M_1T_2F_1S_1ST_3$	T_{93}	$M_2T_1F_1S_1ST_3$	T_{138}	$M_2T_2F_1S_1ST_3$
T_4	$M_1T_1F_1S_1ST_4$	T_{49}	$M_1T_2F_1S_1ST_4$	T_{94}	$M_2T_1F_1S_1ST_4$	T_{139}	$M_2T_2F_1S_1ST_4$
T_5	$M_1T_1F_1S_1ST_5$	T_{50}	$M_1T_2F_1S_2ST_5$	T_{95}	$M_2T_1F_1S_1ST_5$	T_{140}	$M_2T_2F_1S_1ST_5$
T_6	$M_1T_1F_1S_2ST_1$	T_{51}	$M_1T_2F_1S_2ST_1$	T_{96}	$M_2T_1F_1S_2ST_1$	T_{141}	$M_2T_2F_1S_2ST_1$
T_7	$M_1T_1F_1S_2ST_2$	T_{52}	$M_1T_2F_1S_2ST_2$	T_{97}	$M_2T_1F_1S_2ST_2$	T_{142}	$M_2T_2F_1S_2ST_2$
T_8	$M_1T_1F_1S_2ST_3$	T_{53}	$M_1T_2F_1S_2ST_3$	T_{98}	$M_2T_1F_1S_2ST_3$	T_{143}	$M_2T_2F_1S_2ST_3$
T_9	$M_1T_1F_1S_2ST_4$	T_{54}	$M_1T_2F_1S_2ST_4$	T_{99}	$M_2T_1F_1S_2ST_4$	T_{144}	$M_2T_2F_1S_2ST_4$
T_{10}	$M_1T_1F_1S_2ST_5$	T_{55}	$M_1T_2F_1S_2ST_5$	T_{100}	$M_2T_1F_1S_2ST_5$	T_{145}	$M_2T_2F_1S_2ST_5$
T_{11}	$M_1T_1F_1S_3ST_1$	T_{56}	$M_1T_2F_1S_3ST_1$	T_{101}	$M_2T_1F_1S_3ST_1$	T_{146}	$M_2T_2F_1S_3ST_1$
T_{12}	$M_1T_1F_1S_3ST_2$	T_{57}	$M_1T_2F_1S_3ST_2$	T_{102}	$M_2T_1F_1S_3ST_2$	T_{147}	$M_2T_2F_1S_3ST_2$
T_{13}	$M_1T_1F_1S_3ST_3$	T_{58}	$M_1T_2F_1S_3ST_3$	T_{103}	$M_2T_1F_1S_3ST_3$	T_{148}	$M_2T_2F_1S_3ST_3$
T_{14}	$M_1T_1F_1S_3ST_4$	T_{59}	$M_1T_2F_1S_3ST_4$	T_{104}	$M_2T_1F_1S_3ST_4$	T_{149}	$M_2T_2F_1S_3ST_4$
T_{15}	$M_1T_1F_1S_3ST_5$	T_{60}	$M_1T_2F_1S_3ST_5$	T_{105}	$M_2T_1F_1S_3ST_5$	T_{150}	$M_2T_2F_1S_3ST_5$
T_{16}	$M_1T_1F_2S_1ST_1$	T_{61}	$M_1T_2F_2S_1ST_1$	T_{106}	$M_2T_1F_2S_1ST_1$	T_{151}	$M_2T_2F_2S_1ST_2$
T_{17}	$M_1T_1F_2S_1ST_2$	T_{62}	$M_1T_2F_2S_1ST_2$	T_{107}	$M_2T_1F_2S_1ST_2$	T_{152}	$M_2T_2F_2S_1ST_3$
T_{18}	$M_1T_1F_2S_1ST_3$	T_{63}	$M_1T_2F_2S_1ST_3$	T_{108}	$M_2T_1F_2S_1ST_3$	T_{153}	$M_2T_2F_2S_1ST_3$
T_{19}	$M_1T_1F_2S_1ST_4$	T_{64}	$M_1T_2F_2S_1ST_4$	T_{109}	$M_2T_1F_2S_1ST_4$	T_{154}	$M_2T_2F_2S_1ST_4$
T_{20}	$M_1T_1F_2S_1ST_5$	T_{65}	$M_1T_2F_2S_1ST_5$	T_{110}	$M_2T_1F_2S_1ST_5$	T_{155}	$M_2T_2F_2S_1ST_5$
T_{21}	$M_1T_1F_2S_2ST_1$	T_{66}	$M_1T_2F_2S_2ST_1$	T_{111}	$M_2T_1F_2S_2ST_1$	T_{156}	$M_2T_2F_2S_2ST_1$
T_{22}	$M_1T_1F_2S_2ST_2$	T_{67}	$M_1T_2F_2S_2ST_2$	T_{112}	$M_2T_1F_2S_2ST_2$	T_{157}	$M_2T_2F_2S_2ST_2$
T_{23}	$M_1T_1F_2S_2ST_3$	T_{68}	$M_1T_2F_2S_2ST_3$	T_{113}	$M_2T_1F_2S_2ST_3$	T_{158}	$M_2T_2F_2S_2ST_3$
T_{24}	$M_1T_1F_2S_2ST_4$	T_{69}	$M_1T_2F_2S_2ST_4$	T_{114}	$M_2T_1F_2S_2ST_4$	T_{159}	$M_2T_2F_2S_2ST_4$
T_{25}	$M_1T_1F_2S_2ST_5$	T_{70}	$M_1T_2F_2S_2ST_5$	T_{115}	$M_2T_1F_2S_2ST_5$	T_{160}	$M_2T_2F_2S_2ST_5$
T_{26}	$M_1T_1F_2S_3ST_1$	T_{71}	$M_1T_2F_2S_3ST_1$	T_{116}	$M_2T_1F_2S_3ST_1$	T_{161}	$M_2T_2F_2S_3ST_1$
T_{27}	$M_1T_1F_2S_3ST_2$	T_{72}	$M_1T_2F_2S_3ST_2$	T_{117}	$M_2T_1F_2S_3ST_2$	T_{162}	$M_2T_2F_2S_3ST_2$
T_{28}	$M_1T_1F_2S_3ST_3$	T_{73}	$M_1T_2F_2S_3ST_3$	T_{118}	$M_2T_1F_2S_3ST_3$	T_{163}	$M_2T_2F_2S_3ST_1$
T_{29}	$M_1T_1F_2S_3ST_4$	T_{74}	$M_1T_2F_2S_3ST_4$	T_{119}	$M_2T_1F_2S_3ST_4$	T_{164}	$M_2T_2F_2S_3ST_1$
T_{30}	$M_1T_1F_2S_3ST_5$	T_{75}	$M_1T_2F_2S_3ST_5$	T_{120}	$M_2T_1F_2S_3ST_5$	T_{165}	$M_2T_2F_2S_3ST_1$
T_{31}	$M_1T_1F_3S_1ST_1$	T_{76}	$M_1T_2F_3S_1ST_1$	T_{121}	$M_2T_1F_3S_1ST_1$	T_{166}	$M_2T_2F_3S_1ST_1$
T_{32}	$M_1T_1F_3S_1ST_2$	T_{77}	$M_1T_2F_3S_1ST_2$	T_{122}	$M_2T_1F_3S_1ST_2$	T_{167}	$M_2T_2F_3S_1ST_2$
T_{33}	$M_1T_1F_3S_1ST_3$	T_{78}	$M_1T_2F_3S_1ST_3$	T_{123}	$M_2T_1F_3S_1ST_3$	T_{168}	$M_2T_2F_3S_1ST_3$
T_{34}	$M_1T_1F_3S_1ST_4$	T_{79}	$M_1T_2F_3S_1ST_4$	T_{124}	$M_2T_1F_3S_1ST_4$	T_{169}	$M_2T_2F_3S_1ST_4$
T_{35}	$M_1T_1F_3S_1ST_5$	T_{80}	$M_1T_2F_3S_1ST_5$	T_{125}	$M_2T_1F_3S_1ST_5$	T_{170}	$M_2T_2F_3S_1ST_5$
T_{36}	$M_1T_1F_3S_2ST_1$	T_{81}	$M_1T_2F_3S_2ST_1$	T_{126}	$M_2T_1F_3S_2ST_1$	T_{171}	$M_2T_2F_3S_2ST_1$
T_{37}	$M_1T_1F_3S_2ST_2$	T_{82}	$M_1T_2F_3S_2ST_2$	T_{127}	$M_2T_1F_3S_2ST_2$	T_{172}	$M_2T_2F_3S_2ST_2$
T_{38}	$M_1T_1F_3S_2ST_3$	T_{83}	$M_1T_2F_3S_2ST_3$	T_{128}	$M_2T_1F_3S_2ST_3$	T_{173}	$M_2T_2F_3S_2ST_3$
T_{39}	$M_1T_1F_3S_2ST_4$	T_{84}	$M_1T_2F_3S_2ST_4$	T_{129}	$M_2T_1F_3S_2ST_4$	T_{174}	$M_2T_2F_3S_2ST_4$
T_{40}	$M_1T_1F_3S_2ST_5$	T_{85}	$M_1T_2F_3S_2ST_5$	T_{130}	$M_2T_1F_3S_2ST_5$	T_{175}	$M_2T_2F_3S_2ST_5$
T_{41}	$M_1T_1F_3S_3ST_1$	T_{86}	$M_1T_2F_3S_3ST_1$	T_{131}	$M_2T_1F_3S_2ST_1$	T_{176}	$M_2T_2F_3S_3ST_1$
T_{42}	$M_1T_1F_3S_3ST_2$	T_{87}	$M_1T_2F_3S_3ST_2$	T_{132}	$M_2T_1F_3S_3ST_3$	T_{177}	$M_2T_2F_3S_3ST_2$
T_{43}	$M_1T_1F_3S_3ST_3$	T_{88}	$M_1T_2F_3S_3ST_3$	T_{133}	$M_2T_1F_3S_3ST_3$	T_{178}	$M_2T_2F_3S_3ST_3$
T_{44}	$M_1T_1F_3S_3ST_4$	T_{89}	$M_1T_2F_3S_3ST_4$	T_{134}	$M_2T_1F_3S_3ST_3$	T_{179}	$M_2T_2F_3S_3ST_4$
T_{45}	$M_1T_1F_3S_3ST_5$	T_{90}	$M_1T_2F_3S_3ST_5$	T_{135}	$M_2T_1F_3S_3ST_3$	T_{180}	$M_2T_2F_3S_3ST_5$

Table 2 : Effect of vatrious factors on chemical attributes of yoghurt

Factors	Chemical attributes					
	Fat (%)	Protein (%)	Lactose (%)	Ash (%)	Acidity (%)	pH
Sources of milk	Cow milk	5.02	4.72	5.19	1.02	4.55
	Buffalo milk	5.02	4.72	5.32	1.02	4.54
Temperture	39⁰C	5.02	4.72	5.32	1.02	4.57
	42⁰C	5.02	4.72	5.19	1.02	4.52
	4%	4.02	4.71	5.26	1.02	4.55
Fat	5%	5.02	4.72	5.28	1.02	4.55
	6%	6.02	4.72	5.22	1.02	4.54
	10%	5.02	4.29	4.81	0.88	4.60
SNF	11%	5.03	4.67	5.25	0.97	4.53
	12%	5.02	5.19	5.70	1.20	4.51
	Set 1(SL1 : 1)	5.03	4.71	5.19	1.01	4.63
	Set 2 (SL 1 : 2)	5.01	4.73	5.38	1.01	4.61
	Set 3 (SL 1: 3)	5.02	4.71	5.56	1.01	4.59
Starter Culture	Set 4 (SL 2 :1)	5.03	4.72	5.13	1.03	4.47
	Set 5 (SL 3 : 1)	5.01	4.72	5.01	1.02	4.44

Factors	Chemical attributes	CD	
		5%	1%
	Fat	Not significant	
	Protein	Not significant	
Sources of milk	Lactose	0.043	0.057
	Ash	Not singificant	
	Acidity (Lactic acid)	0.004	0.005
	pH	0.007	0.009
	Fat	Not significant	
	Protein	Not significant	
	Lactose	0.043	0.057
Temperature	Ash	Not significant	
	Acidity (Lactic acid)	0.004	0.005
	pH	0.007	0.009
	Fat	0.018	0.023
	Protein	Not significant	
	Lactose	Not significant	
	Ash	Not significant	
Fat	Acidity (Lactic acid)	Not significant	
	pH	0.008	Not significant

SNF	Fat	Not significant	
	Protein	0.020	0.027
	Lactose	0.053	0.069
	Ash	0.014	0.018
	Acidity (Lactic acid)	0.004	0.006
	pH	0.008	0.011
Starter culture	Fat	Not significant	
	Protein	Not significant	
	Lactose	0.068	0.089
	Ash	Not significant	
	Acidity (Lactic acid)	0.006	0.008
	pH	0.011	0.014

8 Results and Discussion

The results obtained during entire investigation (Kumar, 2002) have been discussed into two phases, which are given hereunder:

Phase - I

In this phase of investigation, cow and buffalo milk samples were standardized with three levels of fat and SNF. All the standardized milk samples were treated with five levels of starter culture and incubated at 39°C and 42°C separately for preparation of yoghurt. Thus, the total of 180 treatment combinations were made. Each sample was judged by a panel of five judges to find out the effects of above factors on physical attributes (flavour, body and texture, acidity and colour & appearance) of yoghurt. The samples were also chemically analysed to findout the effect of the same factors on chemical attributes of yoghurt.

The data obtained in this phase of study, were statistically analysed and are presented in the form of table and graphs (wherever necessry). The detail of experimental results obtained are discussed here under :

A. Physical attributes

4.1 The effects of different factors on the physical attributes (flavour, body & texture, acidity and colour & appearance) of yoghurt

4.1.1 Source of milk

A perusal of data presented in the table (Table - 1.0) clearly indicate that the flavour source of yoghurt prepared from cow milk (36.71) was significantly (P < 0.01) higher than the average value found in yoghurt samples prepared from buffalo milk (36.27). When the other physical attributes were compared, the values were significantly (P < 0.01) higher in case of buffalo milk made sample as compared to yoghurt prepared from cow milk. These results clearly indicate that the flavour score is inversely proportion to the score of body & texture, acidity and colour & appearance, irrespective of the source of milk.

The higher flavour score found in yoghurt sample prepared from cow milk might be due to the higher concentration of citric acid in cow milk which is directly related with the flavour production in milk and milk products. The higher body & texture score found in buffalo milk yoghurt sample may be due to presence of higher fat and SNF content in the milk. The rest of the attributes are mostly depends on the liking of the judges. Arjano et al. (1988) and Akin and Konar (1993) reported that the yoghurt made from cow milk received higher flavour quality than that made from goat milk. This result can be compared with the yoghurt prepared from buffalo and cow milk in the present investigation.

4.1.2 Temperature

The score of the body and texture, acidity & colour and appearance were 25.20, 11.29 and 3.72 in the yoghurt sample prepared at 42°C and 24.77, 11.13 and 3.67 in the sample prepared at 39°C, respectively (Table 1.0). The differences in the values obtained at two different incubation temperature were statistically very high (P < 0.01). The increase in the flavour score (16.42%) was very high as compared to the score recorded by body and texture (1.73%), acidity (1.44%) and colour & appearance (1.36%) in yoghurt prepared at 42°C as compared to the values recorded from the sample prepared at 39°C. The higher score of physical attributes in the yoghurt prepared at higher tenperature may be due of favourable growth of bacteria at higher temperature which are directly responsible for the production of good quality yoghurt.

Table 1.0 : The effects of various factors on the physical attributes of yoghurt

Factor		Physical attributes			
		Flavour	Body & texture	Acidity (score)	Colour & appearance
Sources of milk	Cow milk	36.71	24.80	11.17	3.56
	Buffalo milk	36.27	25.16	11.25	3.83
Temperature	39°C	33.72	24.77	11.13	3.67
	42°C	39.26	25.20	11.29	3.72
	4%	34.65	24.71	11.09	3.44
Fat	5%	36.51	25.04	11.21	3.71
	6%	38.31	25.20	11.35	3.94
	10%	35.88	23.28	11.05	3.56
SNF	11%	36.39	24.51	11.21	3.68
	12%	37.19	27.17	11.38	3.85
	Set$_1$ (SL 1 : 1)	36.47	24.78	11.11	3.69
Starter culture	Set$_2$ (SL 1 : 2)	37.18	24.96	11.35	3.69
	Set$_3$ (SL 1 : 3)	39.69	25.94	12.10	3.69
	Set$_4$ (SL 2 : 1)	35.46	24.71	10.86	3.70
	Set$_5$ (SL 3: 1)	33.64	24.53	10.64	3.70

Factors	Physical attributes	CD	
		5%	1%
Sources of milk	Flavour	0.09	0.12
	Body & texture	0.08	0.11
	Acidity (score)	0.05	0.06
	Colour & appearance	0.04	0.05
Temperature	Flavour	0.09	0.12
	Body & texture	0.08	0.11
	Acidity (score)	0.05	0.06
	Colour & appearance	0.04	0.05
Fat	Flavour	0.11	0.15
	Body & texture	0.10	0.13
	Acidity (score)	0.06	0.08
	Colour & appearance	0.04	0.06
SNF	Flavour	0.11	0.15
	Body & texture	0.10	0.13
	Acidity (score)	0.06	0.08
	Colour & appearance	0.04	0.06
Starter culture	Flavour	0.14	0.19
	Body & texture	0.13	0.17
	Acidity (score)	0.08	0.10
	Colour & appearance	Not singificant	

Dolejalek and Vokacova (1981) obtained the best quality yoghurt when the milk sample was incubated at 42°C as compared to yoghurt prepared at lower temperature. This result is directly corroborate with the finding reported by Magdesi (1979), who found that the fermented milk produced from mixture of liquid and reconstituted milk at 36°C had better sensory properties than those coagulated at 42°C.

4.1.2.1 Interaction effects of temperature and sources of milk on physical attributes of yoghurt

Flavour

The flavour score was significantly (P < 0.01) higher in yoghurt samples prepared from cow milk as compared to the values observed from buffalo milk, at both the tenperature (Table-1.1). Further, it was also noted that flavour score increased p<0.01 at 42°c while decreased at 39°c in the sample prepared from buffalo milk. The best flavour score have also been reported by Gono et al. (1988) in cow milk yoghurt prepared at 42°C as compared to the sample obtained at 48°C or 54°C.

Table 1.1 :   The interaction effect of temperature and sources of milk on flavour score of yoghurt

Sources of milk	Temperature	
	T_1 (39°C)	T_2(42°C)
M_1(Cow milk)	33.82	39.59
M_2 (Buffalo milk)	33.62	38.92
Average	33.72	39.26

CD at 5% = 0.13, at 1% =0.17

Body and texture

The body and texture score of yoghurt increased with increase in temperature, irrespective of sources of milk and vice-versa (Table-1.2), but the difference between the values was not significant. The highest body and texture score (25.36) was recorded in the sample prepared from buffalo milk at 42°C incubation temperature, while the sample prepared at 39°C temperature from cow milk scored lowest value (24.57).

Table 1.2 : The interaction effect of temperature and sources of milk on body and texture score of yoghurt

Sources of milk	Temperature	
	T_1 (39°C)	T_2(42°C)
M_1(Cow milk)	24.57	25.04
M_2 (Buffalo milk)	24.97	25.36
Average	24.77	25.20

Acidity score

The interaction effects of temperature and sources of milk did not show any statistical significance on acidity score of yoghurt (Table - 1.3). The acidity score of sample prepared from both kinds of milk at 42°C were the maximum than the acidity score obtained at 39°C.

Table 1.3 : The interaction effects of temperature and sources of milk on acidity score of yoghurt

Sources of milk	Temperature	
	T_1 (39°C)	T_2(42°C)
M_1(Cow milk)	11.10	11.25
M_2 (Buffalo milk)	11.17	11.34
Average	11.13	11.29

Colour and appearance

The differences in the interaction effects of temperature and sources of milk on colour and appearance score of yoghurt did not show any statistical significant (Table - 1.4). The colour and appearance score of buffalo milk yoghurt was higher than the cow milk yoghurt, incubated at both the temperatures.

Table 1.4 :   The interactions effect of temperature and sources
              of milk on colour and appearance score of yoghurt.

Not significant

Sources of milk	Temperature	
	T_1 (39°C)	T_2(42°C)
M_1(Cow milk)	3.54	3.58
M_2 (Buffalo milk)	3.80	3.86
Average	3.67	3.72

4.1.2.2 Interaction effects of temperature and fat on physical attributes of yoghurt

Flavour

A critical observation of the data presented in table-1.5 revealed that the flavour score of yoghurt samples prepared at both the temperature were significantly increased (P < 0.01) as the concentration of fat increases in the milk. The flavour score recorded in interaction groups T_2F_1, T_2F_2, T_2F_3, T_1F_1, T_1F_2 and T_1F_3 were 37.73, 39.30, 40.73, 31.57, 33.72 and 35.88, respectively. The differences in flavour score recorded from yoghurt prepared between two different temperature were very high (P < 0.01). The maximum flavour score (40.73) was recorded in the sample prepared at 42°C in association with 6.0% fat in milk and the minimum value (31.57) was recorded in the sample prepared at 39°C from 4.0% fat.

Table 1.5 :   The interaction effect of temperature and fat on
              flavour score of yoghurt

CD at 5% = 0.16, at 1% = 0.21

Temperature	Fat		
	F_1 (4%)	F_2 (5%)	F_3 (6%)
T_1(39°C)	31.57	33.72	35.88
T_2 (42°C)	37.73	39.30	40.73
Average	34.65	36.51	38.31

Body and texture

The data on body and texture score of yoghurt presented in table-1.6 indicate that body and texture quality of yoghurt prepared at 42°C was improved (P < 0.05) as concentration of fat increased in milk. The average body and texture score was recorded as 24.87, 25.23 and 25.51 in interaction groups T_2F_1, T_2F_2 and T_2F_3, respectively. The score of yoghurt samples prepared at higher temperature were significantly higher (P < 0.05) than the values recorded from the samples prepared at lower temperature. The body and texture score of yoghurt prepared at 42°C increased significantly (P < 0.05) when fat content in milk was increased from 4.0 to 5.0%, but further increase in fat content (5.0 to 6.0%) did not show any significantly increase in the score. The highest and lowest body and texture score were recorded in combination group F_3T_2 and F1T1, respectively.

Table 1.6 :   The interaction effect of temperature and fat on body and texture score of yoghurt

Temperature	Fat		
	F_1 (4%)	F_2 (5%)	F_3 (6%)
T_1 (39°C)	24.54	24.85	24.90
T_2 (42°C)	24.87	25.23	25.51
Average	24.71	25.04	25.20

CD at 5% = 0.14, at 1% = N.S.

Acidity score

The acidity score of yoghurt samples prepared at 39°C in association with different levels of fat were lower than the values recorded from the samples prepared at higher temperature (Table 1.7), but the differences among the values were statistically not significant. The maximum acidity score (11.44) was recorded form the sample prepared at higher incubation temperature with higher level of fat whereas, the minimum value (11.03) was recorded from the sample prepared at lower temperature and fat.

Table 1.7 :   The interaction effect of temperature and fat on acidity score of yoghurt

Temperature	Fat		
	F_1 (4%)	F_2 (5%)	F_3 (6%)
T_1(39°C)	11.03	11.11	11.25
T_2 (42°C)	11.14	11.30	11.44
Average	11.09	11.21	11.35

Not significant

Colour and appearance

At both the incubation temperature, the colour and appearance score of yoghurt was increased with increasing the levels of fat in milk but the differences in the values were statistically not significant (Table - 1.8). The best colour and appearance score (3.96) was shown by the yoghurt sample prepared at 42°C in association with 6.0% fat. Although, this score was at par with the value recorded in yoghurt sample prepared at lower temperature (39°C) with 6.0% fat in milk.

Table 1.8 :   The interaction effect of temperature and fat on colour and appearances score of yoghurt

Temperature	Fat		
	F_1 (4%)	F_2 (5%)	F_3 (6%)
T_1(39°C)	3.41	3.68	3.92
T_2 (42°C)	3.47	3.74	3.96
Average	3.44	3.71	3.94

Not significant

4.1.2.3 Interaction effect of temperature and SNF on physical attributes of yoghurt.

Flavour

The flavour score of yoghurt prepared at 39°C improved significantly ($P < 0.01$) as the concentration of SNF in milk increases (Table - 1.9). The flavour score was recorded as 33.00,

33.67 and 34.50 in interaction groups T_1S_1, T_1S_2 and T_1S_3, respectively. The flavour score recorded from sample prepared at 39°C was significantly lower (P<0.01) than the value recorded from the samples prepared at 42°C, irrespective of SNF levels in milk. The maximum increase (17.48%) in flavour score was observed in T_2S_1 interaction group followed by groups T2S2 (16.19%) and T_2S_3 915.59%) than the value obtained in combination groups T_1S_1, T_1S_2 and T_2S_3, respectively. The flavour was the highest (39.88) in interaction group T_2S_3 and the lowest (33.00) in interaction group T_1S_1.

Table 1.9 : The interaction effect of temperature and SNF flavour score of yoghurt

Temperature	SNF		
	S_1 (4%)	S_2 (5%)	S_3 (6%)
T_1(39°C)	33.00	33.67	34.50
T_2 (42°C)	38.77	39.12	39.88
Average	35.88	36.39	37.19

CD at 5% = 0.16, at 1% = 0.21

Body and texture

It is very clear from the data presented in the table (Table- 2.0) that the body and texture score of yoghurt significantly increased (P<0.01) as the SNF content in milk increases during preparation of yoghurt at 39°C and 42°C. Further, it was also noted that the score recorded from the samples prepared at 42°C with different levels of SNF were significantly higher (P< 0.01) than the score recorded from the samples prepared at lower temperture. The maximum body and texture score (237.48) was recorded in sample prepared at higher temperature in association with higher level of SNF and the minimum value (23.11) was observed in the sample prepared at lower temperature (39°C) in combination with the lower level of SNF.

Table 2.0 :   The interaction effect of temperature and SNF on acidity score of yoghurt

Temperature	SNF		
	S_1 (4%)	S_2 (5%)	S_3 (6%)
T_1(39°C)	23.11	24.33	26.86
T_2 (42°C)	23.45	24.68	27.48
Average	23.28	24.51	27.17

CD at 5% = 0.14, at 1% = 0.18

Acidity score

The acidity score of yoghurt increased with increase of SNF concentration in milk prepared at both the incubation temperature, but the differences in the values were statistically not significant (Table 2.1). The increase or decrease in acidity score of yoghurt as influenced by temperature and SNF were similar as recorded for body & texture score of yoghurt, but the differences in the score were statistically non-significant.

Table 2.1 :   The interaction effect of temperature and SNF on acidity score of yoghurt

Temperature	SNF		
	S_1 (4%)	S_2 (5%)	S_3 (6%)
T_1(39°C)	10.96	11.13	11.31
T_2 (42°C)	11.14	11.29	11.45
Average	11.05	11.21	11.38

Not significant

Colour and appearance

Colour and appearance score of yoghurt was apparently increased when incubation temperature increased from 39°C to 42°C, at all the levels of SNF in milk (Table 2.2). The differences in the values obtained from different interaction groups did not show any statistical significance. The colour and appearance score was also increased at every increase on the levels of SNF in milk at both temperature level. The increase in the colour & apperance of yoghurt between the interaction groups did not show any statistical significance.

Table 2.2 :   The interaction effect of temperature and SNF on colour and appearance score of yoghurt

Temperature	SNF		
	S_1 (4%)	S_2 (5%)	S_3 (6%)
T_1(39°C)	3.53	3.65	3.83
T_2 (42°C)	3.59	3.70	3.87
Average	3.56	3.68	3.85

Not significant

4.1.2.4 Interaction effect of temperature and starter culture on physical quality of yoghurt

Flavour

The data presented in table-2.3 revealed that the flavour score increased significantly (P < 0.01) as the concentration of *lactobacilli* increases in the mixed culture of yoghurt prepared at 39°C, but the values abruptly decreased (P < 0.01) even from the normal level when the levels of streptococci increases in the culture. The flavour score of yoghurt was noted as 33.39, 34.19, 36.86, 32.94 and 31.22 in interaction groups T_1Set_1, T_1Set_2, T_1Set_3 T_1Set_4, and T_1Set_5, respectively. These flavour scores were significantly (P < 0.01) lower than the values recorded from the yoghurt prepared at 42°C, irrespective of the culture used. The minimum flavour score (31.22) was recorded in he yoghurt prepared at 39°C in culture group SL 3: 1 and the maximum value (42.53) was recorded in the sample of culture group SL : 1:3 at 42°C.

Table 2.3 : The interaction effect of temperature and starter culture on flavour score of yoghurt

Temperature	Starter Culture				
	Set_1 (SL 1:1)	Set_2 (SL 1:2)	Set_3 (SL 1: 3)	Set_4 (SL 2 : 1)	Set_5 (SL 3 : 1)
$T_1(39^0C)$	33.39	34.19	36.86	32.94	31.22
$T_2 (42^0C)$	39.56	40.17	42.53	42.53	36.06
Average	36.47	37.18	39.69	39.69	33.64

CD at 5% = 0.20, at 1% = 0.27

Body and texture

The combined effects of temperature and starter culture on body and texture quality of yoghurt were apparently higher in the sample prepared at 42°C than the values recorded in samples prepared at 39°C (Table - 2.4). The increase or decrease in the body and texture score of yoghurt as influenced by temperature and the levels of bacteria were similar as it was recorded form flavour score of yoghurt (Table 2.3), but the differences in the score were statistically not significant.

Table 2.4 : The interaction effect of temperature and starter culture on body and texture score of yoghurt

Temperature	Starter Culture				
	Set_1 (SL 1:1)	Set_2 (SL 1:2)	Set_3 (SL 1: 3)	Set_4 (SL 2 : 1)	Set_5 (SL 3 : 1)
$T_1(39^0C)$	24.57	24.74	25.70	24.49	24.32
$T_2 (42^0C)$	24.99	25.18	26.18	24.92	24.74
Average	24.78	24.96	25.94	24.71	24.53

Not significant

Acidity score

A critical observation of the data given in table - 2.5 show that the interaction effect between temperature and different levels of bacterial culture did not show any statistical significance on acidity score of yoghurt. The best acidity score (12.11) was shown by the yoghurt sample prepared with the highest level of lactobacilli at higher incubation temperature (42°C). Although, this score was at par with the value (12.09) recorded from interaction Set_3 and T_1. The acid score was always higher in yoghurt prepared at 420C, irrespective of the culture used as compared to be values recorded at 39°C. The difference in the values recorded from all intersection groups were statistically not significant.

Table 2.5 : The interaction effect of temperature and starter culture on acidity score of yoghurt

Temperature	Starter Culture				
	Set_1 (SL 1:1)	Set_2 (SL 1:2)	Set_3 (SL 1: 3)	Set_4 (SL 2 : 1)	Set_5 (SL 3 : 1)
T_1(39°C)	11.04	11.29	12.09	10.71	10.53
T_2 (42°C)	11.17	11.41	12.11	11.02	10.76
Average	11.11	11.35	12.10	10.86	10.65

Not significant

Colour and appearance

Colour and appearance of yoghurt prepared at higher incubation temperature were apparently higher than the value recorded at lower temperature, irrespective of the culture used (Table - 2.6). No any definite trend in the colour and appearance score could be identified on increasing or decreasing levels of culture and temperature during manufacture of yoghurt.

Table 2.6 : The interaction effect of temperature and starter culture on colour and appearance score of yoghurt

Temperature	Starter Culture				
	Set_1 (SL 1:1)	Set_2 (SL 1:2)	Set_3 (SL 1: 3)	Set_4 (SL 2 : 1)	Set_5 (SL 3 : 1)
T_1(39°C)	3.67	3.66	3.67	3.67	3.67
T_2 (42°C)	3.72	3.72	3.73	3.72	3.72
Average	3.69	3.69	3.70	3.70	3.70

Not significant

4.1.3 Fat

It is clear from the data presented in table- 1.0 that the average flavour score of yoghurt prepared from 4.0% milk fat was 34.64, which increased simultaneously as the levels of fat increases in the milk. The differences in flavour score of yoghurt prepared at various levels of fat were statistically significant ($P < 0.01$). This increase in the flavour score were 5.36 and 10.56 per cent at increase of 1.0% and 2.0% fat in milk from initial level of 4.0% fat. The similar pattern was also observed in other quality parameters viz., body and texture, acidity and colour and appearance of yoghurt. The score of flavour, body & texture, acidity and colour & appearance were 34.65, 24.71, 11.09 and 3.44 in the samples prepared with 5% fat and 38.31, 25.20, 11.35 and 3.94 in the samples prepared from milk containing 6.0% fat. The differences between the values obtained in each attributes were statistically very high ($P < 0.01$).

By nature, fat is rich in flavour producing compound, diacetyle methyl carbinol, therefore, the increase or decrease in flavour of yoghurt is directly related with amount of fat present in the sample. The reason behind the improvement of body and texture score of yoghurt may be due to increase in the total solids of milk because the body and texture score of fermented milk product is directly related with total solids content of milk whereas, fat is a part of it. The rest of the attributes are mostly depends on the likings of the judges. Similar, results have also been observed by Chawala and Balachandran (1993) and Venkateshaiah et al. (1994) when yoghurt was prepared from different levels of fat present in buffalo milk.

4.1.3.1 Interaction effect of fat and sources of milk on physical attributes of yoghurt

Flavour

The data presented in table- 2.7 indicate that the flavour score of yoghurt increased constantly with increase the fat content of milk prepared from cow and buffalo milk both. The flavour score of M_2F_1 (34.53), M_2F_2 (36.18), and M_2F_3 (38.10), treatment combinations were significantly (P < 0.01) lower the then the values recorded from the treatment combination groups M_1F_1 (34.77), M_1F_2 (36.83) and M_1F_3 (38.52).

Table 2.7 : The interaction effect of fat and sources of milk on flavour score of yoghurt

Sources of milk	Fat		
	F_1 (4%)	F_2(5%)	F_3 (6%)
M_1(Cow milk)	34.77	36.83	38.52
M_2 (Buffalo milk)	34.53	36.18	38.10
Average	34.65	36.51	38.31

CD at 5% = 0.16, at 1% = 0.21

Body and texture

The average body and texture score was recorded as 24.57, 24.89 and 24.95 in interaction groups M_1F_1, M_1F_2 and M_1F_3 and 24.85, 25.19 and 25.46 in interaction groups M_2F_1, M_2F_2 and M_2F_3 respectively (Table - 2.8). These value clearly show that the body and texture score recorded from the yoghurt sample prepared from buffalo milk in association with different levels of fat were significantly (P < 0.05) higher than the value recorded from the sample prepared at the same level of fat in milk. The maximum (25.46). body and texture score was obtained by M_2F_3 treatment, whereas, the lowest (24.57) score was recorded in treatment group M_1F_1. Futher, it was also observed that the body and texture score of yoghurt significantly (P < 0.05) increased as the content of fat in milk increase, irrespective of the sources of milk.

Table 2.8 : The interaction effect of fat and sources of milk on body and texture score of yoghurt

Sources of milk	Fat		
	F_1 (4%)	F_2(5%)	F_3 (6%)
M_1(Cow milk)	24.57	24.89	24.95
M_2 (Buffalo milk)	24.85	25.19	25.46
Average	24.71	24.04	25.20

CD at 5% = 0.14, at 1% = N.S.

Acidity score

The combined effect fat and sources of milk on acidity score of yoghurt prepared from buffalo milk was apparently higher than the value recorded in cow milk yoghurt (Table - 2.9). The increase or decrease in acidity score of samples as influenced by fat and sources of milk were similar to body and texture score of yoghurt (Table - 2.8).

Table 2.9 : The interaction effect of fat and sources of milk on acidity score of yoghurt

Sources of milk	Fat		
	F_1 (4%)	F_2(5%)	F_3 (6%)
M_1(Cow milk)	11.04	11.17	11.31
M_2 (Buffalo milk)	11.13	11.24	11.38
Average	11.09	11.21	11.35

Not significant

Colour and appearance

A critical observation of data presented in table - 3.0 show that the colour and appearance of yoghurt increased significantly ($P < 0.01$) as the concentration of fat increases in buffalo milk. The colour and appearance score was noted as 3.65, 3.81 and 4.04 in interaction group M_2F_1, M_2F_2 and M_2F_3, respectively. These values were significantly ($P < 0.01$) higher than the values recorded from cow milk yoghurt samples. The trend of increase in colour and appearance score of yoghurt, prepared from cow milk, was similar as it was noted in the samples prepared from buffalo milk. The maximum colour and appearance score (4.04) was recorded in the M_2 x F_3 interaction group whereas, the minimum value (3.23) was observed in interaction group M_1 x F_1.

Table 3.0 :   The interaction effect of fat and sources milk on colour and appearance score of yoghurt

Sources of milk	Fat		
	F_1 (4%)	F_2(5%)	F_3 (6%)
M_1(Cow milk)	3.23	3.61	3.84
M_2 (Buffalo milk)	3.65	3.81	3.04
Average	3.44	3.71	3.94

CD at 5% = 0.06, at 1% = 0.08

4.1.3.2 The interaction effect of fat and SNF on physical attributes of yoghurt

Flavour

The flavour score of yoghurt sample increased as the levels of fat and SNF in milk increases (Table 3.1). The average flavors score of the sample as influenced by various levels of fat and SNF groups F_1 S_1, F_1 S_2, F_1 S_3, F_2 S_1, F_2 S_2, F_2 S_3 and F_3 S_1, F_3 S_2, F_3 S_3 were 34.08, 34.58, 35.30, 35.83, 36.43, 37.28 and 37.75, 38.18, 39.00 respectively. The maximum score (39.00) was observed in sample containing higher levels of fat and SNF whereas, the minimum value (34.00) was recorded in sample containing minimum level of fat and SNF. However, the differences in the values were statistically not significant.

Table 3.1 :   The interaction effect of fat and SNF on flavour score of yoghurt

Fat	SNF		
	S_1 (10%)	S_2(11%)	S_3 (12%)
F_1(4%)	34.08	34.58	35.30
F_2 (5%)	35.83	36.43	37.28
F_3 (6%)	37.75	38.18	39.00
Average	35.88	36.39	37.19

Not significant

Body and texture

It is obviously clear from the values presented in table-3.2 that the yoghurt prepared from higher level of fat and SNF in milk sample secured higher body and texture value (27.33) whereas, the lowest value (22.94) was observed in the sample prepared from lowest level of fat and SNF in milk. The differences in the values recorded from different interaction groups were statistically not significant.

Table 3.2 :   The interaction effect of fat and SNF on body and texture score of yoghurt

Fat	SNF		
	S_1 (10%)	S_2(11%)	S_3 (12%)
F_1(4%)	22.94	24.24	26.94
F_2 (5%)	23.32	24.57	27.24
F_3 (6%)	23.57	24.71	27.33
Average	23.28	24.51	27.17

Not significant

Acidity score

The acidity score of yoghurt constantly increased as the concentration of SNF in milk increases, irrespective of fat levels and vice-versa (Table-3.3). The minimum score (10.92) was recorded in yoghurt sample prepared from lower level of fat and SNF. The differences in the values observed from various interaction groups were statistically not significant.

Table 3.3 :   The interaction effect of fat and SNF on acidity score of yoghurt

Fat	SNF		
	S_1 (10%)	S_2(11%)	S_3 (12%)
F_1(4%)	10.92	11.08	11.26
F_2 (5%)	11.05	11.20	11.37
F_3 (6%)	11.19	11.35	11.52
Average	11.05	11.21	11.38

Not significant

Colour and appearance

The colour and appearance score of yoghurt increased significantly (P < 0.01) with increase in the levels of fat in milk, irrespective of levels of SNF in the milk (Table - 3.4). The colour and appearence score for interaction groups $F_1 S_1$, $F_2 S_1$, $F_3 S_1$, $F_1 S_2$, $F_3 S_2$, $F_1 S_3$, $F_2 S_3$ and $F_3 S_3$ were 3.30, 3.60, 3.78, 3.45, 3.73, 3.86, 3.57, 3.80 and 4.19, respectively. The maximum increase (17.37%) in colour and appearance score of yoghurt was observed when concentration of fat and SNF both were the highest. However, the minimum value was observed in interaction groups F1 S1.

Table 3.4 :   The interaction effect of fat and SNF on colour and appearance score of yoghurt

Fat	SNF		
	S_1 (10%)	S_2(11%)	S_3 (12%)
F_1(4%)	3.30	3.45	3.57
F_2 (5%)	3.60	3.73	3.80
F_3 (6%)	3.78	3.86	4.19
Average	3.56	3.68	3.85

CD at 5% = 0.07, at 1% = 0.10

4.1.3.3. The interaction effect of fat and starter culture on physical attributes of yoghurt

Flavour

The data presented in Table 3.5 clearly depict that the flavour of yoghurt increased significantly (P <0.01) as the levels of lactobacilli and fat increases in the milk. It was also observed that the flavour score of yoghurt decreased significantly (P < 0.01) when the proportion of streptococci increase in the culture. It is also notable from the data that as the levels of fat increases in the milk, the flavour score of the product was also increased significantly (P < 0.01), irrespective of bacteria used in the culture. The maximum flavour score (41.67) was recorded in the combination group SL_1 : 3 x F_3, whereas the minimum value (31.83) was recorded in combination group F_1 x SL_3 : 1.

Table 3.5 :   The interaction effect of fat and starter on starter culture on flavour score of yoghurt

Starter culture	Fat		
	F1 (4%)	F2 (5%)	F3 (6%)
Set1 (SL 1 : 1)	34.63	36.33	38.46
Set2 (SL 1 : 2)	35.33	37.17	39.04
Set3 (SL 1 : 3)	37.71	39.71	41.67
Set4 (SL 2 : 1)	33.75	35.46	37.17
Set5 (SL 3 : 1)	31.83	33.88	35.21
Average	34.65	36.51	38.31

CD at 5% = 0.25, 1% = 0.33

Body and texture

A critical observation of the data recorded in table-3.6 revealed that the body and texture of yoghurt samples prepared form milk containing 4.0% and 5.0% fat were apparently increased when the concentration of lactobacilli was doubled in the mixed culture. As the concentration of lactobacilli enchanced thrice in the milk containing 4.0 and 5.0% fat, the body & texture of yoghurt increased significantly ($P < 0.05$). In case of yoghurt prepared from milk containing 6% fat the body and texture score increased significantly ($P < 0.05$) as the levels of lactobacilli increases in the culture. It was also noted that body & texture quality of the samples apparently reduced when the yoghurt was prepared with increasing levels of streptococci in the milk containing 4% and 5% fat. The body and texture of the samples reduced significantly ($P < 0.05$) when yoghurt was prepared with milk containing 6% fat and triple concentration of streptococci.

Table 3.6 : The interaction effect of fat and starter culture on body and texture score of yoghurt

Starter culture	Fat		
	F1 (4%)	F2 (5%)	F3 (6%)
Set1 (SL 1 : 1)	24.54	24.80	25.00
Set2 (SL 1 : 2)	24.70	24.97	25.22
Set3 (SL 1 : 3)	25.50	25.99	26.33
Set4 (SL 2 : 1)	24.48	24.79	24.85
Set5 (SL 3 : 1)	24.32	24.66	24.61
Average	24.71	24.04	25.20

CD at 5% = 0.22, at 1% = N.S.

The body and texture of yoghurt was also improved (P < 0.05) with increasing the content fat in milk, irrespective of levels of starter culture used. The increase in the textural quality of yoghurt was not significant when the concentration of fat increased from 5.0 to 6.0% in milk fermented with cultures S L 1 : 1, SL 2 : 1 and SL 3 : 1 culture.

Acidity score

The data presented in Table 3.7 clearly indicate that on increasing the levels of fat and sterptococci in the mixed culture the acidity score of samples enhanced. The differences in the values obtained between the interaction groups were statistically not significant.

Table 3.7 : The interaction effect of fat and starter culture on acidity score of yoghurt

Starter culture	Fat		
	F1 (4%)	F2 (5%)	F3 (6%)
Set1 (SL 1 : 1)	10.93	11.11	11.28
Set2 (SL 1 : 2)	11.26	11.32	11.47
Set3 (SL 1 : 3)	11.90	12.08	12.33
Set4 (SL 2 : 1)	10.75	10.88	10.97
Set5 (SL 3 : 1)	10.58	10.65	10.70
Average	11.09	11.21	11.35

Not significant

Colour and appearance

The colour and appearance score of yoghurt improved as the concentration of fat increases in milk, irrespective of starter culture used (Table - 3.8). However, increasing the lactobacilli and sterptococci in the starter culture did not affect the colour and appearance of yoghurt prepared at all the levels of fat.

Table 3.8 :   The interaction effect of fat and starter culture on colour and appearance score of yoghurt

Starter culture	Fat		
	F1 (4%)	F2 (5%)	F3 (6%)
Set1 (SL 1 : 1)	3.43	3.71	3.94
Set2 (SL 1 : 2)	3.43	3.71	3.94
Set3 (SL 1 : 3)	3.44	3.70	3.94
Set4 (SL 2 : 1)	3.43	3.72	3.94
Set5 (SL 3 : 1)	3.45	3.70	3.95
Average	3.44	3.71	3.94

Not significant

4.1.4 SNF

A perusal of the data presented in table - 1.0 clearly indicate that the yoghurt prepared from milk containing 12% SNF scored significantly ($P < 0.01$) higher flavour than the sample prepared from 10 and 11% SNF. A significant ($P < 0.01$) increase in the score was also noted for body & texture, acidity and colour & appearance of yoghurt samples prepared from increased levels of SNF. At the increase of 1% SNF (from 10 to 11%) the body texture gained 5.28% but the score gained thrice, when the level of SNF increased from 10 to 12 percent. For colour appearance the increase was noted as 3.37% and 8.15%, for flavour 1.42% and 3.65% and for acidity 1.45% and 3.00% on increased the levels of SNF from, 10 to 11% and 10 to 12%, respectively. These increase on the physical attributes of yoghurt were stastistically very high ($P < 0.01$).

Significantly constant improvement in the body and texture of yoghurt might be due to increase of the total solids in milk.

Rasic and Kurman (1982) have reported that body and texture of fermented products may increase with increasing the concentration of SNF in the milk. Citric acid is a precurser of flavour producing compound (diacetyl) in fermented milk porducts. This might be reason behing the increases in the milk. Rasic and Kurman (1982), Banks and Evans (1983), Ritcher et al. (1979) and Becker and Puhan (1989) also reported similar effect of SNF on physical attributes of yoghurt prepared from skim milk or cow milk or buffalo milk.

4.1.4.1. Interaction effects of SNF and sources of milk on physical attributes of yoghurt

Flavour

The Flavour of yoghurt prepared from cow and buffalo milk both, apparently increased with increasing the levels of SNF in milk (Table - 3.9). The flavour of cow milk youghurt was higher as compresed to the value recolded from from buffalo milk samples, at all the levels of SNF included in the milk. The differences in the flavour score did not show any statistical significance. The minimum score (35.67) was recorded in yoghurt sample prepared from buffalo milk having 10.0% SNF and the maximum value (37.40) was recorded in cow milk yoghurt containing 12.0% SNF.

Table 3.9 :   The interaction effect of SNF and source of milk flavour score of yoghurt.

Sources of milk	SNF		
	S_1 (10%)	S_2(11%)	S_3 (12%)
M_1(Cow milk)	36.10	36.62	37.40
M_2 (Buffalo milk)	35.67	36.17	36.98
Average	35.88	36.39	37.19

Not significant

Body and texture

The body and texture quality of cow and buffalo milk yoghurt was singificantly ($P < 0.01$) improved with increasing the levels of SNF in milk (Table 4.0). The average score were noted as 23.38, 24.68 and 27.44 in interaction groups M_2S_1, M_2S2, and M_2S_3, respectively. These values were significantly (P < 0.01) higher than the value recorded from M_1 S_1, M_1 S_2 and M_1S_3 interaction groups. The peak value (27.44) was recorded in sample prepared from the highest level of SNF in buffalo milk, whereas the sample prepared from lower level of SNF in cow milk scored the lowest value. (23.18).

Table 4.0 :   The interaction effect of SNF and sources of milk on body and texture score of yoghurt

Sources of milk	SNF		
	S_1 (10%)	S_2(11%)	S_3 (12%)
M_1(Cow milk)	23.18	24.33	26.91
M_2 (Buffalo milk)	23.38	24.68	27.44
Average	23.28	24.51	27.17

CD at 5% = 0.14, at 1% = 0.18

Acidity score

The increase or decrease in the acidity score of yoghurt (Table - 4.1) as influenced by the SNF in both type of milk were at par as it was recorded for body and texture score of yoghurt (tabke-4.0), but the differences in the values were not significant. The maximum value (11.42) was recorded in M_2S_3 interaction group and the minimum score (11.00) was noted in interaction group M_1 S_1.

Table 4.1 :   The interaction effect of SNF and sources of milk on acidity score of yoghurt

Sources of milk	SNF		
	S_1 (10%)	S_2(11%)	S_3 (12%)
M_1(Cow milk)	11.00	11.18	11.34
M_2 (Buffalo milk)	11.10	11.23	11.42
Average	11.05	11.21	11.38

Not significant

Colour and appearance

The data given in the table (Table 4.2) clearly depict that the colour and appearance of yoghurt was apparently improved as the concentration of SNF increases in milk, irrespective of the sources of milk. The highest colour and appearance score (4.01) was recorded in combination group M_2 x S_3 whereas, the lowest score (3.42) was recorded in group M_1 x S_1.

Table 4.2 :   The interaction effect of SNF and sources of milk on colour and appearance score of yoghurt

Sources of milk	SNF		
	S_1 (10%)	S_2(11%)	S_3 (12%)
M_1(Cow milk)	3.42	3.56	3.69
M_2 (Buffalo milk)	3.70	3.79	4.01
Average	3.56	3.68	3.85

Not significant

4.1.4.2. Interaction effect of SNF and starter culture on physical attributes of yoghurt

Flavour

It can be seen from the table (Table -4.3) that the observed values in respect of flavour score of yoghurt were 35.79 (Set$_1$ S$_1$), 36.58 (Set$_2$ S$_1$), 39.17 (Set$_3$ S$_1$), 34.88 (Set$_4$ S$_1$), 33.00 (Set$_5$ S$_1$), 36.4 (Set$_1$ S$_2$), 37.13 (Set$_2$ S$_2$), 40.42 (Set$_3$ S$_3$), 36.17 (Set$_4$ S$_3$) and 34.38 (Set$_5$ S$_3$). The maximum flavour score was observed in group S$_3$ Set$_3$ whereas, S$_1$ Set$_5$ group scored very least value. The flavour of yoghurt constantly increased with increase in levels of SNF, irrespective of bacterial culture used. It was also observed that as the proportions of lactobacilli enhanced for coagulation of milk, the flavour of the sample also increases, but differences in the values were statistically not significant. The flavour quality of yoghurt sample apparently reduced as the proportion of streptococci increases in the sample.

Table 4.3 :　The interaction effect of SNF and starter culture on flavour score of yoghurt

Starter culture	SNF		
	S_1 (10%)	S_2 (11%)	S_3 (12%)
Set$_1$ (SL 1: 1)	35.79	36.46	37.17
Set$_2$ (SL 1: 2)	36.58	37.13	37.83
Set$_3$ (SL 1 : 3)	39.17	39.50	40.42
Set$_4$ (SL 2 : 1)	34.88	35.33	36.17
Set$_5$ (SL 3 : 1)	33.00	33.54	34.38
Average	35.88	36.39	37.19

Not significant

Body and texture

A critical observation of data presented in table - 4.4 indicate that the body and texture quality of yoghurt improved significantly ($P < 0.01$) as the concentration of SNF increases in milk, irrespective of bacteria used in starter culture. When bacterial concentration in the culture were taken into account, the score of body and texture improved significantly ($P < 0.01$) as the proportion of lactobacilli increased to three fold at all the levels of SNF in milk used. The body and texture in the yoghurt also improved when the level of lactobacilli was doubled in the milk containing 10%, 11% and 12% levels of SNF, but the differences in the values were statistically insignificant. It was also notable from the data that the body and texture score of yoghurt reduced significantly ($P < 0.01$) at double and triple levels of streptococci used in the milk containing 10% SNF. The difference in values found in the Set$_4$ and Set$_5$ was statistically not significant. Other effects of culture and SNF did not show any statistically significance.

Table 4.4 : The interaction effect of SNF and starter culture on body and texture score of yoghurt

Starter culture	SNF		
	S_1 (10%)	S_2 (11%)	S_3 (12%)
Set$_1$ (SL 1: 1)	22.87	24.46	27.02
Set$_2$ (SL 1: 2)	23.04	24.64	27.20
Set$_3$ (SL 1 : 3)	24.08	25.42	28.33
Set$_4$ (SL 2 : 1)	23.28	24.09	26.79
Set$_5$ (SL 3 : 1)	23.12	23.93	26.54
Average	23.28	24.51	27.17

CD at 5% = 0.22, at 1% = 0.29

Acidity Score

On increasing the levels of SNF in milk, the acidity score of yoghurt apparently increased, irrespective of the levels of starter culture used. The maximum acidity score (12.38) was recorded in sample prepared from 12.0% SNF in milk with culture group SL 1 : 3 and the minimum value (10.52) was observed in sample prepared from the lowest SNF (10.0%) with culture group SL 3 : 1.

Table 4.5 : The interaction effect of SNF and starter culture on acidity score of yoghurt

Starter culture	SNF		
	S_1 (10%)	S_2 (11%)	S_3 (12%)
Set$_1$ (SL 1: 1)	10.96	11.11	11.26
Set$_2$ (SL 1: 2)	11.20	11.33	11.51
Set$_3$ (SL 1 : 3)	11.84	12.08	12.38
Set$_4$ (SL 2 : 1)	10.73	10.86	11.00
Set$_5$ (SL 3 : 1)	10.52	10.65	10.77
Average	11.05	11.21	11.38

Not significant

Colour and appearance

The data presented in table - 4.6 clearly indicate that the colour and apparance score of yoghurt apparently increased with increasing the concentration of SNF in milk, irrespective of starter culture used. However, increasing or decreasing of lactobacilli and streptococci in the starter culture did not show any significant impact on colour and appearance of yoghurt at any level of SNF added in the milk.

Table 4.6 :   The interaction effect of SNF and starter culture on colour and appearance score of yoghurt

Starter culture	SNF		
	S_1 (10%)	S_2 (11%)	S_3 (12%)
Set_1 (SL 1: 1)	3.56	3.68	3.85
Set_2 (SL 1: 2)	3.56	3.68	3.85
Set_3 (SL 1 : 3)	3.56	3.68	3.85
Set_4 (SL 2 : 1)	3.55	3.68	3.86
Set_5 (SL 3 : 1)	3.58	3.68	3.85
Average	3.56	3.68	3.85

Not significant

4.1.5 Starter culture

A critical observation of data presented in table - 1.0. Clearly show that all the physical attributes, except colour and appearance of yoghurt, significant ($P < 0.01$) increased as the levels of *L. bulgaricus* increases in the starter culture, but the same was not true when the proportion of *S. thermophillus* enhanced in the culture. These physical attributes were decreased significantly ($P < 0.01$) as the levels of streptococci increases in the culture and vice-versa. However, increasing or decreasing the concentration of these two bacteria in the culture did not affect the colour and appearance score of yoghurt. The increase (8.91%) in acidity score was comparatively very high than the increase in flavour (8.83%) and body and texture (4.68%) score of yoghurt, when concentration of lactobacilli increased three fold in the starter culture than the normal one (SL 1 : 1).

The increase in the flavour score of yoghurt prepared with increasing the levels of *L.bulgaricus* bacteria in culture may be due to the fact the that the *L. bulgaricus* bacteria produces flavour and acid both whereas, the *S. thermophilus* produces acids only.

Therefore, samples prepared with the starter culture containing higher concentration of lactobacilli had (P < 0.01) higher flavour than the samples prepared with higher level of streptococci. Galestoot et al. (1968), Moon and Reinbold (1978), Shankar and Davis (1976), Lal et al. (1978), Chawla and Balchandran (1985) and Klic (1986) made yoghurt of desired sensory characteristics by using *S. thermophilus* and *L. bulgaricus* strain in the ratio of 1 : 1 which is directly corroborate with the finding of present study. The improvement in the quality of yoghurt has also been reported by Lal et al. (1978) and Kilic (1986) when the ratios of *L bulgaricus* increases in the culture which is in agreement with the results obtained in the present study.

4.1.5.1 Interaction effect of starter culture and sources of milk on physical attributes of yoghurt

Flavour

It is clear from the data shown in table- 4.7 that on increasing the levels of lactobacilli in the culture, the flavour of yoghurt increased significantly (P < 0.01) whereas, the trend was reversed (P < 0.01) when levels of S. thermophillus enhanced in the culture, irrespective the type of milk used. The cow milk yoghurt prepared with all the levels of culture had significantly (P < 0.01) better flavour than the sample prepared with all the same level of culture used in buffalo milk, except the group M1 Set_4 (35.31) and the group M_2Set_4 (35.61). The interaction effect of starter culture M_2 Set_4 in cow milk sample was significantly lower than the flavour score observed in M_2Set_5 (33.20). A contradictory results to our findings was reported by Singh and Kaul, who found good flavour in yoghurt prepared by buffalo milk than cow milk sample.

Table 4.7 : The interaction effect of starter culture and sources of milk on flavour score of yoghurt

Sources of milk	Starter culture				
	Set$_1$ (SL 1 : 1)	Set$_2$ (SL 1 : 2)	Set$_3$ (SL 1 : 3)	Set$_4$ (SL 2: 3)	Set$_5$ (SL 3 : 1)
M$_1$ (Cow milk)	36.86	37.44	39.92	35.31	34.00
M$_2$ Buffalo milk)	36.08	36.92	39.47	35.61	33.28
Average	36.47	37.18	39.69	35.46	33.64

CD at 5% = 0.20, at 1% = 0.27

Body and texture

The body and texture of cow and buffalo milk yoghurt was increased as the concentration of lactobacilli increases in the culture, but the effect of increasing levels of streptococci in the culture were reverse. The differences in the values for body and texture score of buffalo milk yoghurt samples prepared with various levels of starter culture were comparatively higher than the cow milk yoghurt, but the differences among the values were statistically not significant. The lowest score (24.64) was observed in interaction group M$_1$Set$_1$ whereas, the highest score (26.14) was recorded in interaction group M$_2$Set$_3$.

Table 4.8 :   The interaction effect of starter culture and sources of milk on body & texture of yoghurt

Sources of milk	Starter culture				
	Set$_1$ (SL 1 : 1)	Set$_2$ (SL 1 : 2)	Set$_3$ (SL 1 : 3)	Set$_4$ (SL 2: 3)	Set$_5$ (SL 3 : 1)
M$_1$ (Cow milk)	24.64	24.82	25.74	24.51	24.31
M$_2$ Buffalo milk)	24.92	25.10	26.14	24.91	24.75
Average	24.78	24.96	25.94	24.71	24.53

Not significant

Acidity score

The increase in the acidity score was directly related with increasing in the concentration of lactobacilli in cow and buffalo milk yoghurt both. The differences in the values obtained from different interaction groups did not show any statistical significance (Table 4.9).

Table 4.9 : The interaction effect of starter culture and sources of milk on acidity score of yoghurt

Sources of milk	Starter culture				
	Set$_1$ (SL 1 : 1)	Set$_2$ (SL 1 : 2)	Set$_3$ (SL 1 : 3)	Set$_4$ (SL 2: 3)	Set$_5$ (SL 3 : 1)
M$_1$ (Cow milk)	11.07	11.28	12.04	10.87	10.60
M$_2$ Buffalo milk)	11.14	11.41	12.16	10.86	10.69
Average	11.11	11.35	12.10	10.86	10.64

Not significant

Colour and appearance

It is clear from the data presented in the table (Table- 5.0) that on increasing or decreasing the concentration of lactobacilli and streptococci in the starter culture did not affect the colour and appearance scope of yoghurt prepared from cow or buffalo milk. Colour and appearance score of buffalo milk yoghurt samples were apparently higher than the cow milk yoghurt samples prepared with all the levels of starter culture used for coagulation of milk.

Table 5.0 : The interaction effect of starter culture and sources of milk on colour & appearance score of yoghurt

Sources of milk	Starter culture				
	Set$_1$ (SL 1 : 1)	Set$_2$ (SL 1 : 2)	Set$_3$ (SL 1 : 3)	Set$_4$ (SL 2: 3)	Set$_5$ (SL 3 : 1)
M$_1$ (Cow milk)	3.56	3.55	3.56	3.55	3.57
M$_2$ Buffalo milk)	3.83	3.83	3.83	3.84	3.83
Average	3.69	3.69	3.69	3.70	3.70

Not significant

4.1.6 : Interaction effect of temperature, sources of milk and fat on physical attributes of yoghurt

Flavour

The data presented in the table (Table 5.1) indicate that the flavour quality of yoghurt prepared from cow and buffalo milk, improved significantly (p<0.01) as content of fat was enhenced in milk at both incubation temperature. The flavour of both milk (M_1 & M_2) yoghurt was also improved significantly (P < 0.01) when its incubation temperature increased from 39 to 42°C, irrespective of fat levels. The score of yoghurt samples prepared from cow and buffalo milk, at 42°C incubation temperature with various levels of fat were significantly (P < 0.01) higher as compared to the score obtained from the samples prepared at 39°C with same level fat. When flavour of cow milk yoghurt sample were compared with buffalo milk yoghurt, the cow milk yoghurt proved to have better flavour quality than the buffalo milk yoghurt.

Table 5.1 : The interaction effect of temperature, sources of milk and fat on flavour score of yoghurt

Fat	Sources of milk x Temperature			
	M_1 (Cow milk)		M_2 (Buffalo milk)	
	T_1 (39°C)	T_2 (42°C)	T_1 (39°C)	T_2 (42°C)
F_1(4%)	31.57	37.97	31.57	37.50
F_2 (5%)	33.80	39.87	33.63	38.73
F_3 (6%)	36.10	40.93	35.67	40.53
Average	33.82	39.59	33.62	38.92

CD at 5% = 0.22, CD at 1% = 0.29

The interaction effect of temperature, sources of milk and fat on body & texture, acidity score and colour & appearance of yoghurt were statistically not significant (Table 5.2, 5.3 and 5.4).

Table 5.2 : The interaction effect of temperature, sources of milk and fat levels on body and texture score of yoghurt

Fat	Sources of milk x Temperature			
	M_1 (Cow milk)		M_2 (Buffalo milk)	
	T_1 (39°C)	T_2 (42°C)	T_1 (39°C)	T_2 (42°C)
F_1(4%)	24.39	24.75	24.70	24.99
F_2 (5%)	24.72	25.07	24.99	25.39
F_3 (6%)	24.58	25.31	25.22	25.70
Average	24.57	24.04	24.97	25.36

Not significant

Table 5.3 : The interaction effect of temperature, sources of milk and fat levels on acidity score of yoghurt

Fat	Sources of milk x Temperature			
	M_1 (Cow milk)		M_2 (Buffalo milk)	
	T_1 (39°C)	T_2 (42°C)	T_1 (39°C)	T_2 (42°C)
F_1(4%)	10.98	11.10	11.09	11.17
F_2 (5%)	11.07	11.27	11.16	11.33
F_3 (6%)	11.25	11.37	11.25	11.51
Average	11.10	11.25	11.17	11.34

Not significant

Table 5.4 : The interaction effect of temperature, sources of milk and fat levels on colour and appearance score of yoghurt

Fat	Sources of milk x Temperature			
	M_1 (Cow milk)		M_2 (Buffalo milk)	
	T_1 (39°C)	T_2 (42°C)	T_1 (39°C)	T_2 (42°C)
F_1(4%)	3.21	3.25	3.61	3.68
F_2 (5%)	3.58	3.63	3.78	3.84
F_3 (6%)	3.83	3.85	4.02	4.07
Average	3.54	3.58	3.80	3.86

Not significant

4.1.7 : Interaction effect of temperature, sources of milk and SNF on physical attributes of yoghurt

Flavour

The data presented in table - 5.5 clearly indicate that the flavour quality of yoghurt, prepared from cow and buffalo milk, significantly ($P < 0.01$) improved as the levels of incubation temperature increases, irrespective of SNF level in milk. The flavour quality of cow and buffalo milk yoghurt also enhanced with enhanced levels of SNF in milk at incubation temperature of 39°C and 42°C. The flavour score of yoghurt prepared from buffalo milk was significantly ($P < 0.01$) lower than the score obtained from cow milk yoghurt. The value of interaction groups $M_1T_1S_1$ and $M_2T_1S_1$ were the same.

Table 5.5 : The interaction effect of temperature, sources of milk and SNF on flavour score of yoghurt

SNF	Sources of milk x Temperature			
	M_1 (Cow milk)		M_2 (Buffalo milk)	
	T_1 (39°C)	T_2 (42°C)	T_1 (39°C)	T_2 (42°C)
S_1(10%)	33.00	39.20	33.00	38.33
S_2 (11%)	33.80	39.43	33.53	38.80
S_3 (12%)	34.67	40.13	34.33	39.63
Average	33.82	39.59	33.62	38.92

CD at 5% = 0.22, CD at 1% = 0.29

Body and texture

The textural quality of yoghurt prepared from cow and buffalo milk at 39°C and 42°C incubation temperature improved significantly ($P < 0.01$) as the concentration of SNF increases in the milk (Table 5.6). Textural quality of yoghurt samples, prepared from buffalo milk in association with different levels of SNF and incubation temperature, were significantly ($P < 0.01$) superior to the textural quality of yoghurt samples prepared from cow milk in association with the same level of SNF and incubation temperature.

The cow milk yoghurt prepared at lower temperature with the lowest level of SNF had least (23.03) textural score whereas, the highest textural score (27.59) was recorded in the buffalo milk yoghurt prepared at higher level of incubation temperature with the highest level of SNF in milk.

Table 5.6 : The interaction effect of temperature, sources of milk and SNF on body and texture score of yoghurt

SNF	Sources of milk x Temperature			
	M_1 (Cow milk)		M_2 (Buffalo milk)	
	T_1 (39°C)	T_2 (42°C)	T_1 (39°C)	T_2 (42°C)
S_1(10%)	23.03	23.33	23.19	23.57
S_2 (11%)	24.23	24.44	24.44	24.93
S_3 (12%)	26.44	27.37	27.28	27.59
Average	24.57	25.04	24.97	25.36

CD at 5% = 0.02, CD at 1% = 0.26

The interaction effect of temperature, sources of milk and SNF on acidity score (Table 5.7) and colour & appearance (Table - 5.8) quality of yoghurt were not significant.

Table 5.7 : The interaction effect of temperature, sources of milk and SNF on acidity score of yoghurt

SNF	Sources of milk x Temperature			
	M_1 (Cow milk)		M_2 (Buffalo milk)	
	T_1 (39°C)	T_2 (42°C)	T_1 (39°C)	T_2 (42°C)
S_1(10%)	10.61	11.08	11.01	11.20
S_2 (11%)	11.11	11.25	11.15	11.32
S_3 (12%)	11.28	11.41	11.35	11.49
Average	11.10	11.25	11.14	11.34

Not significant

Table 5.8 : The interaction effect of temperature, sources of milk and SNF on colour and appearance score of yoghurt

SNF	Sources of milk x Temperature			
	M_1 (Cow milk)		M_2 (Buffalo milk)	
	T_1 (39°C)	T_2 (42°C)	T_1 (39°C)	T_2 (42°C)
S_1(10%)	3.40	3.45	3.66	3.74
S2 (11%)	3.55	3.58	3.76	3.82
S_3 (12%)	3.67	3.71	3.99	4.03
Average	3.54	3.58	3.80	3.86

Not significant

4.1.8 : The interaction effect of temperature, sources of milk and starter culture on physical attributes of yoghurt

Flavour

The data presented in table - 5.9 clearly depict that the flavour of yoghurt enhanced significantly (P < 0.01) with increasing the concentration of lactobacilli irrespective of temperature and type of milk (cow and buffalo) used, but when the concentration of streptococci increases in the milk, the flavour quality of yoghurt reduced significantly (P < 0.01). The flavour quality of yoghurt prepared form cow and buffalo milk also improved significantly (P < 0.01) as the levels of temperature increases, irrespective of starter culture used. The combined effect of milk, temperature and starter culture of flavour was significantly higher in yoghurt sample prepared from cow milk than the yoghurt smaples obtained from buffalo milk. The highest flavour score (42.94) was noted in interaction group M_1 x T_3 x Set_3 and the lowest (30.78) was recorded in interaction group M_2 x T_1 x Set_5.

Table 5.9 : The interaction effect of temperature, sources of milk and starter culture on flavour score of yoghurt

| Starter culture | Sources of milk x Temperature | | | |
| | M_1 (Cow milk) | | M_2 (Buffalo milk) | |
	T_1 (39°C)	T_2 (42°C)	T_1 (39°C)	T_2 (42°C)
Set$_1$ (SL 1:1)	33.61	40.11	33.17	39.00
Set$_2$ (SL 1:2)	34.22	40.67	34.17	39.67
Set$_3$ (SL 1:3)	36.89	42.94	36.83	42.11
Set$_4$ (SL 2:3)	32.72	37.89	33.17	38.06
Set$_5$ (SL 3:1)	31.67	36.33	33.78	35.78
Average	33.82	39.59	33.62	38.92

CD at 5% = 0.29, CD at 1% = 0.38

The interaction effects of temperature, sources of milk and starter culture on body and texture, acidity score and colour and appearance of yoghurt were not significant. (Table - 6.0 and 6.2).

Table 6.0 : The interaction effect of temperature, sources of milk and starter culture on body and texture score of yoghurt

Not significant

| Starter culture | Sources of milk x Temperature | | | |
| | M_1 (Cow milk) | | M_2 (Buffalo milk) | |
	T_1 (39°C)	T_2 (42°C)	T_1 (39°C)	T_2 (42°C)
Set$_1$ (SL 1:1)	24.43	24.86	24.71	25.13
Set$_2$ (SL 1:2)	24.62	25.02	24.87	25.33
Set$_3$ (SL 1:3)	25.57	25.92	25.83	26.44
Set$_4$ (SL 2:3)	24.20	24.81	24.79	25.03
Set$_5$ (SL 3:1)	24.01	24.61	24.63	24.87
Average	24.57	24.05	24.97	25.36

Acidity

The data presented in table-6.1 clearly show that the acidity score of yoghurt significantly ($P < 0.01$) increased with increasing concentration of lactobacilli in the culture irrespective of temperature of sources of milk, whereas increasing the concentration of streptococci significantly (P < 0.01) reduces the acidity score prepared at both levels of temperature and milk. Though the differences in the value of interaction groups $M_1T_2Set_1$ and $M_1T_2Set_4$ and $M_2T_1Set_5$, $M_1T_1Set_1$ and $M_1T_2Set_1$, $M_1T_1Set_2$ and $M_1T_2Set_2$ & M_2T_2Set1 were statistically insignificant.

Table 6.1 : The interaction effect of temperature, sources of milk and starter culture on acidity score of yoghurt.

Starter culture	Sources of milk x Temperature			
	M1 (Cow milk)		M2 (Buffalo milk)	
	T1 (39°C)	T2 (42°C)	T1 (39°C)	T2 (42°C)
Set$_1$ (SL 1:1)	10.99	11.16	11.10	11.19
Set$_2$ (SL 1:2)	11.21	11.36	11.67	11.46
Set$_3$ (SL 1:3)	12.16	11.39	12.02	12.29
Set$_4$ (SL 2:3)	10.68	11.06	10.74	10.98
Set$_5$ (SL 3:1)	10.47	10.73	10.60	10.78
Average	11.10	11.25	11.14	11.34

CD at 5% = 0.16, CD at 1% = 0.21

Table 6.2 : The interaction effect of temperature, sources of milk and starter culture on colour and appearance score of yoghurt

Starter culture	Sources of milk x Temperature			
	M_1 (Cow milk)		M_2 (Buffalo milk)	
	T_1 (39°C)	T_2 (42°C)	T_1 (39°C)	T_2 (42°C)
Set$_1$ (SL 1:1)	3.53	3.58	3.80	3.86
Set$_2$ (SL 1:2)	3.52	3.59	3.80	3.86
Set$_3$ (SL 1:3)	3.52	3.59	3.80	3.86
Set$_4$ (SL 2:3)	3.54	3.56	3.80	3.87
Set$_5$ (SL 3:1)	3.57	3.58	3.81	3.86
Average	3.54	3.58	3.80	3.86

Not significant

4.1.9 Interaction effect of temperature, fat and SNF on physical attributes of yoghurt

The flavour (table - 6.3), body & texture (table - 6.5) and colour & appearance (table 6.6) quality of yoghurt, apprently increased at increasing levels of fat, SNF and temperature of milk during preparation of sample.

Table 6.3 : The interaction effect of temperature, fat and SNF on flavour score of yoghurt

SNF	Temperature x Fat					
	T_1 (39^{0}C)			T_2 (42^{0}C)		
	F_1 (4%)	F_2 (5%)	F_3 (6%)	F_4 (4%)	F_5 (5%)	F_6 (6%)
S_1 (10%)	30.85	33.05	35.10	37.30	38.60	40.40
S_2 (11%)	31.55	33.60	35.85	37.60	39.25	40.50
S_3 (12%)	32.30	34.50	36.70	38.30	40.05	41.30
Average	31.57	33.72	35.88	37.73	39.30	40.73

Not significant

Table 6.4 : The interaction effect of temperature, fat and SNF on body and texture score of yoghurt

SNF	Temperature x Fat					
	T_1 (39^{0}C)			T_2 (42^{0}C)		
	F_1 (4%)	F_2 (5%)	F_3 (6%)	F_4 (4%)	F_5 (5%)	F_6 (6%)
S_1 (10%)	22.79	23.16	23.37	23.10	23.48	23.76
S_2 (11%)	24.21	24.37	24.42	24.28	24.76	25.01
S_3 (12%)	26.64	27.03	26.92	27.24	27.45	27.75
Average	24.54	24.85	24.90	24.87	25.23	25.51

Not significant

Table 6.5 : The interaction effect of temperature, fat and SNF
             on acidity score of yoghurt

SNF	Temperature x Fat					
	T_1 (39°C)			T_2 (42°C)		
	F_1 (4%)	F_2 (5%)	F_3 (6%)	F_4 (4%)	F_5 (5%)	F_6 (6%)
S_1 (10%)	10.85	10.95	11.08	10.99	11.14	11.29
S_2 (11%)	11.02	11.11	11.25	11.13	11.29	11.44
S_3 (12%)	11.23	11.28	11.43	11.29	11.46	11.60
Average	11.03	11.11	11.25	11.14	11.30	11.44

Not significant

Table 6.6 : The interaction effect of temperature, fat and SNF
             on colour and appearance score of yoghurt

SNF	Temperature x Fat					
	T_1 (39°C)			T_2 (42°C)		
	F_1 (4%)	F_2 (5%)	F_3 (6%)	F_4 (4%)	F_5 (5%)	F_6 (6%)
S_1 (10%)	3.26	3.58	3.75	3.35	3.63	3.81
S_2 (11%)	3.42	3.69	3.85	3.47	3.76	3.88
S_3 (12%)	3.54	3.77	4.17	3.59	3.82	4.20
Average	3.41	3.68	3.92	3.47	3.74	3.96

Not significant

4.1.10 : Interaction effect of temperature, fat, and starter culture
on physical attributes of yoghurt

Flavour

The flavour score of yoghurt increased significantly (P < 0.01)
as the content of fat increases in the milk., irrespective of culture
and temperature used (Table 6.7). The flavour quality of yoghurt
also improved (P < 0.01) when concentration of lactobacilli
increases in the culture at all the levels of fat and incubation
temperature whereas, the flavour quality of yoghurt reduced
significantly (P < 0.01) as the proportion of streptococci
increases in the culture. The flavour score obtained by yoghurt
samples prepared at lower temperature (39°C) in association

with the various levels of fat and starter culture. The maximum flavour score (43.75) was obtained with higher levels of temperature (42°C) and fat (6%) in association with SL 1:3 culture group. The lowest value (29.58) was obtained when 4.0% fat and culture group SL 3 :1 was put together at 39°C temperature.

Table 6.7 : The interaction effect of temperature, fat and starter culture on flavour score of yoghurt

Starter culture	Temperature x Fat					
	T_1 (39°C)			T_2 (42°C)		
	F_1 (4%)	F_2 (5%)	F_3 (6%)	F_4 (4%)	F_5 (5%)	F_6 (6%)
Set_1 (SL 1:1)	31.17	33.25	35.75	38.08	39.42	41.17
Set_2 (SL 1:2)	32.00	34.08	36.50	38.67	40.25	41.58
Set_3 (SL 1:3)	34.17	36.83	39.58	41.25	42.58	43.75
Set_4 (SL 2:1)	30.92	32.92	35.00	36.58	38.00	39.33
Set_5 (SL 3:1)	29.58	31.50	32.58	34.08	36.25	37.83
Average	31.57	33.72	35.88	37.73	39.30	40.73

CD at 5% = 0.35 at 1% = 0.47

The interaction effect of temperature, fat and starter culture on body and texture (Table - 6.8), acidity score (Table-6.9) and colour & appearance (Table-7.0) of yoghurt were statistically not significant.

Table 6.8 : The interaction effect of temperature, fat and starter culture on acidity score of yoghurt

Starter culture	Temperature x Fat					
	T_1 (39°C)			T_2 (42°C)		
	F_1 (4%)	F_2 (5%)	F_3 (6%)	F_4 (4%)	F_5 (5%)	F_6 (6%)
Set_1 (SL 1:1)	10.85	11.05	11.23	11.02	11.17	11.33
Set_2 (SL 1:2)	11.27	11.23	11.37	11.25	11.40	11.57
Set_3 (SL 1:3)	11.90	12.03	12.33	11.90	12.12	12.32
Set_4 (SL 2:1)	10.63	10.70	10.80	10.87	11.05	11.13
Set_5 (SL 3:1)	10.52	10.55	10.53	10.65	10.75	10.87
Average	11.03	11.11	11.25	11.14	11.30	11.44

Not significant

Table 6.9 : The interaction effect of temperature, fat and starter culture on colour and appearance score of yoghurt

Starter culture	Temperature x Fat					
	T_1 (39°C)			T_2 (42°C)		
	F_1 (4%)	F_2 (5%)	F_3 (6%)	F_4 (4%)	F_5 (5%)	F_6 (6%)
Set₁ (SL 1:1)	3.39	3.69	3.92	3.48	3.73	3.96
Set₂ (SL 1:2)	3.39	3.68	3.92	3.48	3.74	3.96
Set₃ (SL 1:3)	3.40	3.67	3.92	3.48	3.74	3.96
Set₄ (SL 2:1)	3.41	3.69	3.92	3.45	3.74	3.96
Set₅ (SL 3:1)	3.44	3.68	3.94	3.47	3.73	3.96
Average	3.41	3.68	3.92	3.47	3.74	3.96

Not significant

4.1.11 Interaction effect of temperature, SNF and starter culture on physical attributes of yoghurt

The interaction effect of temperature, SNF and starter culture on flavour (Table 7.1), body & texture (Table 7.2), acidity score (Table 7.3) and colour & appearance (Table 7.4) quality of yoghurt were not significant.

Table 7.0 : The interaction effect of temperature, SNF and starter culture on flavour score of yoghurt

Starter culture	Temperature x SNF					
	T_1 (39°C)			T_2 (42°C)		
	S_1 (10%)	S_2 (11%)	S_3 (12%)	S_1 (10%)	S_2 (11%)	S_3 (12%)
Set₁ (SL 1:1)	32.58	33.42	34.17	39.00	39.50	40.17
Set₂ (SL 1:2)	33.42	34.17	35.00	39.75	40.08	40.67
Set₃ (SL 1:3)	36.08	36.75	37.75	42.25	42.25	43.08
Set₄ (SL 2:1)	32.25	32.83	33.75	37.50	37.83	38.58
Set₅ (SL 3:1)	30.67	31.17	31.83	35.33	35.92	36.92
Average	33.00	33.67	34.50	38.77	39.12	39.88

Not significant

Table 7.1 : The interaction effect of temperature, SNF and starter culture on body and texture score of yoghurt.

Starter culture	Temperature x SNF					
	T_1 (39°C)			T_2 (42°C)		
	S_1 (10%)	S_2 11%)	S_3 12%)	S_1 (10%)	S_2 11%)	S_3 12%)
Set$_1$ (SL 1:1)	22.65	24.22	26.84	23.08	24.70	27.20
Set$_2$ (SL 1:2)	22.83	24.41	26.99	23.25	24.7	27.42
Set$_3$ (SL 1:3)	23.87	25.20	28.03	24.28	25.64	28.62
Set$_4$ (SL 2:1)	23.15	23.98	26.35	23.40	24.20	27.17
Set$_5$ (SL 3:1)	23.03	23.85	26.08	23.22	24.00	27.00
Average	23.11	24.33	26.86	23.45	24.68	27.48

Not significant

Table 7.2 : The interaction effect of temperature, SNF and starter culture on acidity score of yoghurt.

Starter culture	Temperature x SNF					
	T_1 (39°C)			T_2 (42°C)		
	S_1 (10%)	S_2 11%)	S_3 12%)	S_1 (10%)	S_2 11%)	S_3 12%)
Set$_1$ (SL 1:1)	10.88	11.05	11.20	11.03	11.17	11.32
Set$_2$ (SL 1:2)	11.12	11.27	11.48	11.28	11.40	11.53
Set$_3$ (SL 1:3)	11.85	12.07	12.35	11.83	12.10	12.40
Set$_4$ (SL 2:1)	10.57	10.70	10.87	10.90	11.02	11.13
Set$_5$ (SL 3:1)	10.38	10.55	10.67	10.65	10.75	10.87
Average	10.96	11.13	11.31	11.14	11.29	11.45

Not significant

Table 7.3 : The interaction effect of temperature, SNF and starter culture on colour and appearance score of yoghurt.

Starter culture	Temperature x SNF					
	T_1 (39°C)			T_2 (42°C)		
	S_1 (10%)	S_2 11%)	S_3 12%)	S_1 (10%)	S_2 11%)	S_3 12%)
Set$_1$ (SL 1:1)	3.53	3.65	3.82	3.59	3.70	3.88
Set$_2$ (SL 1:2)	3.52	3.65	3.82	3.59	3.70	3.88
Set$_3$ (SL 1:3)	3.52	3.65	3.82	3.59	3.71	3.88
Set$_4$ (SL 2:1)	3.52	3.67	3.83	3.58	3.70	3.88
Set$_5$ (SL 3:1)	3.56	3.65	3.85	3.60	3.70	3.85
Average	3.53	3.65	3.83	3.59	3.70	3.87

Not significant

4.1.12 : Interaction effect of fat, sources of milk and SNF on physical attributes of yoghurt

Body and texture

The data presented in table-7.6 clearly indicate that the textural quality of cow and buffalo milk yoghurt enhanced significantly (P < 0.05) as the concentration of fat increases in the milk, at all the levels of SNF in milk. Though the difference in the values of interaction groups $M_1F_2S_1$ & $M_1F_3S^1$, $M_1F_1S_2$ & $M_1F_2S_1$, $M_1F_2S_1$ & $M_1F_3S_1$, $M_1F_2S_2$ & $M_1F_3S_3$ and $M_2F_2S_2$ & $M_2F_3S_2$ were statistically not significant. It was further noted that the body and texture quality of yoghurt improved (P < 0.05) as the content of SNF increases in the milk, irrespective of the levels of fat in milk.

Colour and appearance

The colour and appearance of yoghurt prepared from cow and buffalo milk both increased significantly (P < 0.01) with increasing the concentration of fat in the milk, irrespective of the levels of SNF (Table- 7.8) in milk. Further, it was also noted that the colour and appearance of cow and bufflo milk yoghurt improved (P < 0.01) when the concentration of SNF increased from 10 to 12% in the milk, at all the levels of fat. The differences in the values obtained between interaction groups $M_1F^1S^1$, & $M_1F_1S_2$, $M_1F_2S_1$ & $M_1F_2S_2$, $M_1F_3S_2$ & $M_1F_3S_3$, $M_2F_1S_3$, $M_2F_2S_2$ and $M_2F_3S_2$ & $M_2F_3S_3$ were significant (P < 0.01) whereas, rest of the values did not show any statistical significance.

The score values for flavour (Table-7.5) and acidity (Table - 7.7) did not influenced by the combined effect of fat, sources of milk (cow & buffalo) and SNF.

Table 7.4 : The interaction effect of fat, sources of milk and SNF on flavour and appearance score of yoghurt

SNF	Sources of milk x Fat					
	M₁ (Cow milk)			M₂ (Buffalo milk)		
	F₁ (4%)	F₂ (5%)	F₃ (6%)	F₁ (4%)	F₂ (5%)	F₃ (6%)
S₁ (10%)	34.10	36.20	38.00	34.05	35.45	37.50
S₂ (11%)	34.75	36.75	38.35	34.40	36.10	38.00
S₃ (12%)	35.45	37.55	39.20	35.15	37.00	38.80
Average	34.77	36.83	38.52	34.53	36.18	38.10

Not significant

Table 7.5 : The interaction effect of fat, sources of milk and SNF on body and texture score of yoghurt

SNF	Sources of milk x Fat					
	M₁ (Cow milk)			M₂ (Buffalo milk)		
	F₁ (4%)	F₂ (5%)	F₃ (6%)	F₁ (4%)	F₂ (5%)	F₃ (6%)
S₁ (10%)	34.10	36.20	38.00	34.05	35.45	37.50
S₂ (11%)	34.75	36.75	38.35	34.40	36.10	38.00
S₃ (12%)	35.45	37.55	39.20	35.15	37.00	38.80
Average	34.77	36.83	38.52	34.53	36.18	38.10

CD at 5% = 0.24, at 1% = N.S.

Table 7.6 : The interaction effect of fat, sources of milk and SNF on acidity score of yoghurt

SNF	Sources of milk x Fat					
	M₁ (Cow milk)			M₂ (Buffalo milk)		
	F₁ (4%)	F₂ (5%)	F₃ (6%)	F₁ (4%)	F₂ (5%)	F₃ (6%)
S₁ (10%)	10.86	10.99	11.14	10.8	11.10	11.23
S₂ (11%)	11.05	11.18	11.31	11.10	11.22	11.38
S₃ (12%)	11.21	11.33	11.49	11.31	11.41	11.054
Average	11.04	11.17	11.31	11.13	11.24	11.38

Not significant

Table 7.7 :   The interaction effect of fat, sources of milk and
              SNF on colour and appearance score of yoghurt

SNF	Sources of milk x Fat					
	M_1 (Cow milk)			M_2 (Buffalo milk)		
	F_1 (4%)	F_2 (5%)	F_3 (6%)	F_1 (4%)	F_2 (5%)	F_3 (6%)
S_1 (10%)	3.06	3.49	3.72	3.55	3.72	3.83
S_2 (11%)	3.27	3.62	3.80	3.62	3.83	3.93
S_3 (12%)	3.36	3.71	4.00	3.77	3.88	4.37
Average	3.23	3.61	3.84	3.65	3.84	4.04

CD at 5% = 0.11, at 1% = 0.14

4.1.13 The interaction effect of fat, sources of milk and starter
culture on physical attributes of yoghurt

Flavour

The flavour quality of cow and buffalo milk yoghurt significantly
($P < 0.05$) improved as the content of fat in milk increases,
irrespective of starter culture used (Table-7.9). It was further
noted that the flavour of yoghurt enhanced ($P < 0.05$) when the
proportion of lactobacilli increases in the culture prepared from
cow and buffalo milk both. When the concentration of
streptococci increased in the culture, the combined effect of
fat, sources of milk and starter culture on flavour score of buffalo
milk yoghurt was significantly ($P < 0.05$) lower than the sample
obtained from cow milk. The highest flavour score (41.67) was
observed in interaction group M_1 x F_3 x Set_3 and M_2 x F_3 x Set3
whereas, the lowest value (31.58) was recorded in interaction
group M_2 x F_1 x Set_5.

Table 7.8 : The interaction effect of fat, sources of milk ad starter culture on flavour score of yoghurt

Starter Culture	Sources of milk x Fat					
	M_1 (Cow milk)			M_2 (Buffalo milk)		
	F_1 (4%)	F_2 (5%)	F_3 (6%)	F_1 (4%)	F_2 (5%)	F_3 (6%)
Set_1 (SL 1:1)	34.92	36.75	38.92	34.33	35.92	38.00
Set_2 (SL 1:2)	35.42	37.58	39.33	35.25	36.75	38.75
Set_3 (SL 1:3)	37.83	40.25	41.67	37.58	39.17	41.67
Set_4 (SL 2:1)	33.58	35.33	37.00	33.92	35.58	37.33
Set_5 (SL 3:1)	32.08	34.25	35.67	31.58	33.50	34.75
Average	34.77	36.83	38.52	34.53	36.18	38.10

CD at 5% = 0.35, at 1% = N.S.

The interaction effects of fat, sources of milk and starter culture on body & texture, acidity score and colour & appearance of yoghurt were not significant (Table-8.0, 8.1 and 8.2)

Table 7.9 : The interaction effect of fat, sources of milk and starter culture on body and texture score of yoghurt

Starter Culture	Sources of milk x Fat					
	M_1 (Cow milk)			M_2 (Buffalo milk)		
	F_1 (4%)	F_2 (5%)	F_3 (6%)	F_1 (4%)	F_2 (5%)	F_3 (6%)
Set_1 (SL 1:1)	24.43	24.67	24.83	24.65	24.93	25.18
Set_2 (SL 1:2)	24.60	24.82	25.05	24.79	25.12	25.39
Set_3 (SL 1:3)	25.33	25.78	26.12	25.67	26.20	26.55
Set_4 (SL 2:1)	24.33	24.65	24.53	24.63	24.93	25.17
Set_5 (SL 3:1)	24.16	24.55	24.22	24.48	24.77	25.00
Average	24.57	24.89	24.95	24.85	25.19	25.46

Not significant

Table 8.0 : The interaction effect of fat, sources of milk and starter culture on acidity score of yoghurt

| Starter Culture | Sources of milk x Fat | | | | | |
| | M₁ (Cow milk) | | | M₂ (Buffalo milk) | | |
	F_1 (4%)	F_2 (5%)	F_3 (6%)	F_1 (4%)	F_2 (5%)	F_3 (6%)
Set₁ (SL 1:1)	10.90	11.08	11.23	10.97	11.13	11.33
Set₂ (SL 1:2)	11.17	11.27	11.42	11.35	11.37	11.52
Set₃ (SL 1:3)	11.83	12.00	12.30	11.97	12.15	12.35
Set₄ (SL 2:1)	10.73	10.88	10.98	10.77	10.87	10.95
Set₅ (SL 3:1)	10.57	10.60	10.63	10.60	10.70	10.77
Average	11.04	11.17	11.31	11.13	11.24	11.38

Not significant

Table 8.1 : The interaction effect of fat, sources of milk and starter culture on colour and appearance score of yoghurt

| Starter Culture | Sources of milk x Fat | | | | | |
| | M₁ (Cow milk) | | | M₂ (Buffalo milk) | | |
	F_1 (4%)	F_2 (5%)	F_3 (6%)	F_1 (4%)	F_2 (5%)	F_3 (6%)
Set₁ (SL 1:1)	3.22	3.62	3.84	3.65	3.81	4.03
Set₂ (SL 1:2)	3.22	3.60	3.84	3.65	3.81	4.03
Set₃ (SL 1:3)	3.23	3.59	3.84	3.64	3.82	4.03
Set₄ (SL 2:1)	3.22	3.62	3.83	3.64	3.92	4.05
Set₅ (SL 3:1)	3.27	3.61	3.84	3.64	3.79	4.06
Average	3.23	3.61	3.84	3.65	3.81	4.04

Not significant

4.1.14 Interaction effects of fat, SNF and starter culture on physical attributes of yoghurt

The interaction effect of above factors on physical attributes of yoghurt (Table 8.3, 8.4, 8.5 and 8.6) were statistically not significant.

Table 8.2 :   The interaction effect of fat, SNF and starter culture on flavour score of yoghurt

Starter Culture	Fat x SNF								
	S_1 (10%)	S_2 (11%)	S_3 (12%)	S_1 (10%)	S_2 (11%)	S_3 (12%)	S_1 (10%)	S_2 (11%)	S_3 (12%)
Set$_1$ (SL 1:1)	34.00	34.63	35.25	35.63	36.25	37.13	37.75	38.50	39.13
Set$_2$ (SL 1:2)	34.75	35.25	36.00	36.50	37.13	37.88	38.50	39.00	39.63
Set$_3$ (SL 1:3)	37.13	37.50	38.50	39.13	39.63	40.38	41.25	41.38	42.38
Set$_4$ (SL 2:1)	33.13	33.63	34.50	34.75	35.38	36.25	36.75	37.00	37.75
Set$_5$ (SL 3:1)	31.38	31.88	32.25	33.13	33.75	34.75	34.50	35.00	36.13
Average	34.08	34.58	35.30	35.83	36.43	37.28	37.75	38.18	39.00

Not significant

Table 8.3 :   The interaction effect of fat, SNF and starter culture on body and texture score of yoghurt

Starter culture	Fat x SNF								
	F1 (4%)			F2 (5%)			F3 (6%)		
	S_1 (10%)	S_2 (11%)	S_3 (12%)	S_1 (10%)	S_2 (11%)	S_3 (12%)	S_1 (10%)	S_2 (11%)	S_3 (12%)
Set$_1$ (SL 1:1)	22.65	24.20	26.78	22.90	24.50	27.00	23.05	24.68	27.29
Set$_2$ (SL 1:2)	22.85	24.30	26.94	23.03	24.70	27.18	23.25	24.91	27.50
Set$_3$ (SL 1:3)	23.35	25.09	28.05	24.23	25.53	28.23	24.65	25.65	28.70
Set$_4$ (SL 2:1)	22.98	23.90	26.58	23.30	24.10	26.98	23.55	24.28	26.73
Set$_5$ (SL 3:1)	22.90	23.73	26.35	23.15	24.00	26.83	23.33	24.05	26.45
Average	24.94	24.24	26.94	23.32	24.57	27.24	23.57	24.71	27.33

Not significant

Table 8.4 :   The interaction effect of fat, SNF and starter culture on acidity score of yoghurt

Starter culture	Fat x SNF								
	F1 (4%)			F2 (5%)			F3 (6%)		
	S_1 (10%)	S_2 (11%)	S_3 (12%)	S_1 (10%)	S_2 (11%)	S_3 (12%)	S_1 (10%)	S_2 (11%)	S_3 (12%)
Set$_1$ (SL 1:1)	10.80	10.93	11.08	10.95	11.10	11.28	11.13	11.30	11.43
Set$_2$ (SL 1:2)	11.08	11.23	11.48	11.20	11.33	11.43	11.33	11.45	11.63
Set$_3$ (SL 1:3)	11.65	11.90	12.15	11.80	12.03	12.40	12.08	12.33	12.58
Set$_4$ (SL 2:1)	10.63	10.73	10.90	10.75	10.88	11.00	10.83	10.98	11.10
Set$_5$ (SL 3:1)	10.45	10.60	10.70	10.53	10.68	10.75	10.58	10.68	10.85
Average	10.92	11.08	11.26	11.05	11.20	11.37	11.19	11.35	11.52

Not significant

Table 8.5 : The interaction effect of fat, SNF and starter culture on colour and appearance score of yoghurt

Starter culture	Fat x SNF								
	F1 (4%)			F2 (5%)			F3 (6%)		
	S_1 (10%)	S_2 (11%)	S_3 (12%)	S_1 (10%)	S_2 (11%)	S_3 (12%)	S_1 (10%)	S_2 (11%)	S_3 (12%)
Set₁ (SL 1:1)	3.30	3.4	3.56	3.61	3.73	3.80	3.78	3.86	4.18
Set₂ (SL 1:2)	3.30	3.44	3.56	3.59	3.73	3.80	3.78	3.86	4.18
Set₃ (SL 1:3)	3.28	3.46	3.58	3.61	3.71	3.79	3.78	3.86	4.18
Set₄ (SL 2:1)	3.30	3.43	3.56	3.59	3.76	3.80	3.75	3.86	4.20
Set₅ (SL 3:1)	3.34	3.46	3.56	3.61	3.70	3.79	3.79	3.87	4.20
Average	3.30	3.45	3.57	3.60	3.73	3.80	3.78	3.86	4.19

Not significant

4.1.15 Interaction effect of SNF, sources of milk and starter culture on physical attributes of yoghurt

Body and texture

A critical observation of data presented in table-8.8 indicate that the body and texture quality of yoghurt, prepared from cow and buffalo milk, increased with increase levels of SNF in milk, irrespective of the culture used. When bacterial concentrationin the culture were taken into account, the body and texture score of cow and buffalo milk yoghurt improved significantly ($P < 0.05$) as the proportion of lactobacilli increased to three fold (from 1:1 to 1:2) in the culture, irresoective of the levels of SNF in milk. Although, the body and texture of yoghurt prepared at all the levels of SNF in both and texture of yoghurt prepared at all the levels of SNF in both the milk, improved when the level of lactobacilli was doubled, but the differences in the values were statistically not significant. It was also observed that the body and texture of yoghurt improved ($P < 0.05$) at double and tripled levels of sterptococci in the culture for the sample prepared at 10% level of SNF in cow milk. The body and texture quality of yoghurt improved ($P < 0.05$) when the levels of streptococci was doubled in the culture used in buffalo milk containing 10% SNF. Other effects of SNF, milk and starter culture on body & texture score of yoghurt did not show any statistical significance.

The interaction effect of SNF, sources of milk and starter culture on the score of flavour, acidity and colour & appearance of yoghurt were not significant (Table 8.7, 8.9 and 9.0).

Table 8.6 : The interaction effect of SNF, sources of milk and starter culture on flavour score of yoghurt

Starter culture	Sources of milk x SNF					
	M_1 (Cow milk)			M_2 (Baffalo milk)		
	S_1 (10%)	S_2 (11%)	S_3 (11%)	S_1 (10%)	S_2 (11%)	S_3 (11%)
Set$_1$ (SL 1:1)	36.17	36.83	37.58	35.42	36.08	36.75
Set$_2$ (SL 1:2)	36.83	37.33	38.17	36.33	36.92	37.50
Set$_3$ (SL 1:3)	39.42	39.75	40.58	38.92	39.25	40.25
Set$_4$ (SL 2:1)	34.75	35.25	35.92	35.00	35.42	36.42
Set$_5$ (SL 3:1)	33.33	33.92	34.75	32.67	33.17	34.00
Average	36.10	36.62	37.40	35.67	36.17	36.98

Not significant

Table 8.7 : The interaction effect of SNF, sources of milk and starter culture on body and texture score of yoghurt

Starter culture	Sources of milk x SNF					
	M_1 (Cow milk)			M_2 (Baffalo milk)		
	S_1 (10%)	S_2 (11%)	S_3 (11%)	S_1 (10%)	S_2 (11%)	S_3 (11%)
Set$_1$ (SL 1:1)	22.73	24.27	26.93	23.00	24.65	27.12
Set$_2$ (SL 1:2)	22.93	24.45	27.08	23.15	24.83	27.33
Set$_3$ (SL 1:3)	23.97	25.14	28.12	24.18	25.70	28.53
Set$_4$ (SL 2:1)	23.18	24.00	26.33	23.37	24.18	27.18
Set$_5$ (SL 3:1)	23.06	23.80	26.07	23.18	24.05	27.02
Average	23.18	24.33	26.91	23.38	24.68	27.44

CD at 5% = 0.31, at 1% = N.S.

Table 8.8 : The interaction effect of SNF, sources of milk and
             starter culture on acidity score of yoghurt

Starter culture	Sources of milk x SNF					
	M$_1$ (Cow milk)			M$_2$ (Baffalo milk)		
	S$_1$ (10%)	S$_2$ (11%)	S$_3$ (11%)	S$_1$ (10%)	S$_2$ (11%)	S$_3$ (11%)
Set$_1$ (SL 1:1)	10.90	11.08	11.23	11.02	11.13	11.28
Set$_2$ (SL 1:2)	11.15	11.30	11.40	11.25	11.37	11.62
Set$_3$ (SL 1:3)	11.77	12.03	12.33	11.92	12.13	12.42
Set$_4$ (SL 2:1)	10.72	10.87	11.02	10.75	10.85	10.98
Set$_5$ (SL 3:1)	10.45	10.62	10.73	10.58	10.68	10.80
Average	11.00	11.18	11.34	11.10	11.23	11.42

Not significant

Table 8.9 : The interaction effect of SNF source of milk and
             starter culture on colour and appearance score of
             yoghurt

Starter culture	Sources of milk x SNF					
	M$_1$ (Cow milk)			M$_2$ (Baffalo milk)		
	S$_1$ (10%)	S$_2$ (11%)	S$_3$ (11%)	S$_1$ (10%)	S$_2$ (11%)	S$_3$ (11%)
Set$_1$ (SL 1:1)	3.43	3.56	3.69	3.70	3.79	4.00
Set$_2$ (SL 1:2)	3.41	3.56	3.69	3.70	3.79	4.00
Set$_3$ (SL 1:3)	3.43	3.57	3.68	3.68	3.79	4.02
Set$_4$ (SL 2:1)	3.41	3.56	3.69	3.68	3.81	4.02
Set$_5$ (SL 3:1)	3.44	3.58	3.70	3.72	3.78	4.00
Average	3.42	3.56	3.69	3.70	3.79	4.01

Not significant

4.1.16 Interaction effects of temperature, milk, fat and SNF on
physical attributes of yoghurt

The interaction effects of temperature, milk, fat and SNF on
physical attributes of yoghurt were not significant (Table-9.1,
9.2, 9.3 and 9.4).

Table 9.0 : The interaction effect of temperature, sources of milk, fat and SNF on flavour score yoghurt

SNF	Source of milk x Temperature x Fat											
	M_1 (cow milk)						M_2 (buffalo milk)					
	T_1 (39°C)			T_2 (42 °C)			T_1 (39 °C)			T_2 (42 °C)		
	F_1 (4%)	F_2 (5%)	F_3 (6%)	F_1 (4%)	F_2 (5%)	F_3 (6%)	F_1 (4%)	F_2 (5%)	F_3 (6%)	F_1 (4%)	F_2 (5%)	F_3 (6%)
S_1 (10%)	30.70	33.10	35.20	37.50	39.30	40.80	31.00	33.00	35.00	37.10	37.90	40.00
S_2 (10%)	31.60	33.70	36.10	37.90	39.80	40.60	31.50	33.50	35.60	37.30	38.70	40.40
S_3 (11%)	32.40	34.60	37.00	38.50	40.50	41.40	32.20	34.40	36.40	38.10	39.60	41.20
Average	31.57	33.80	36.10	37.97	39.87	40.93	31.57	33.63	35.67	37.50	38.73	40.53

Not significant

Table 9.1 : The interaction effect of temperature, sources of milk, fat and SNF on body and texture of yoghurt

SNF	Source of milk x Temperature x Fat											
	M_1 (cow milk)						M_2 (buffalo milk)					
	T_1 (39°C)			T_2 (42 °C)			T_1 (39 °C)			T_2 (42 °C)		
	F_1 (4%)	F_2 (5%)	F_3 (6%)	F_1 (4%)	F_2 (5%)	F_3 (6%)	F_1 (4%)	F_2 (5%)	F_3 (6%)	F_1 (4%)	F_2 (5%)	F_3 (6%)
S_1 (10%)	22.74	23.08	23.26	23.08	23.40	23.50	22.84	23.24	23.48	23.12	23.56	24.02
S_2 (10%)	24.20	24.22	24.26	24.01	24.44	24.86	24.22	24.52	24.57	24.54	25.08	25.16
S_3 (11%)	26.24	26.86	26.23	27.16	27.36	27.58	27.03	27.20	27.60	27.32	27.54	27.92
Average	24.39	24.72	24.58	24.75	25.07	25.31	24.70	24.99	25.22	24.99	25.39	25.70

Not significant

Table 9.2 :   The interaction effect of temperature, sources of milk, fat and SNF on acidity score of yoghurt

	Source of milk x Temperature x Fat											
	M_1 (cow milk)						M_2 (buffalo milk)					
	T_1 (39°C)			T_2 (42 °C)			T_1 (39 °C)			T_2 (42 °C)		
SNF	F_1 (4%)	F_2 (5%)	F_3 (6%)	F_1 (4%)	F_2 (5%)	F_3 (6%)	F_1 (4%)	F_2 (5%)	F_3 (6%)	F_1 (4%)	F_2 (5%)	F_3 (6%)
S_1(10%)	10.78	10.88	11.08	10.94	11.10	11.20	10.92	11.02	11.08	11.04	11.18	11.38
S_2(10%)	10.98	11.10	11.24	11.12	11.26	11.38	11.06	11.12	11.26	11.14	11.32	11.50
S_3(11%)	11.18	11.22	11.44	11.24	11.44	11.54	11.28	11.34	11.42	11.34	11.48	11.66
Average	10.98	11.07	11.25	11.10	11.27	11.37	11.09	11.16	11.25	11.17	11.33	11.51

Not significant

Table 9.3 :   The interaction effect of temperature, sources of milk, fat and SNF on colour and appearance score of yoghurt

	Source of milk x Temperature x Fat											
	M_1 (cow milk)						M_2 (buffalo milk)					
	T_1 (39°C)			T_2 (42 °C)			T_1 (39 °C)			T_2 (42 °C)		
SNF	F_1 (4%)	F_2 (5%)	F_3 (6%)	F_1 (4%)	F_2 (5%)	F_3 (6%)	F_1 (4%)	F_2 (5%)	F_3 (6%)	F_1 (4%)	F_2 (5%)	F_3 (6%)
S_1 (10%)	3.04	3.48	3.68	3.08	3.50	3.76	3.48	3.68	3.81	3.61	3.75	3.85
S_2 (10%)	3.26	3.58	3.80	3.28	3.66	3.80	3.58	3.80	3.90	3.66	3.86	3.95
S_3 (11%)	3.32	3.68	4.00	3.40	3.74	4.00	3.76	3.86	4.34	3.78	3.90	4.40
Average	3.21	3.58	3.83	3.25	3.63	3.85	3.61	3.78	4.02	3.68	3.84	4.07

Not significant

Table 9.4 :   The interaction effect of temperature, sources of milk, fat and starter culture on flavour on score of yoghurt

	Source of milk x Temperature x Fat											
	M_1 (cow milk)						M_2 (buffalo milk)					
Starter culture	T_1 (39°C)			T_2 (42 °C)			T_1 (39 °C)			T_2 (42 °C)		
	F_1 (4%)	F_2 (5%)	F_3 (6%)	F_1 (4%)	F_2 (5%)	F_3 (6%)	F_1 (4%)	F_2 (5%)	F_3 (6%)	F_1 (4%)	F_2 (5%)	F_3 (6%)
Set_1 (SL 1:1)	31.33	33.33	36.17	38.50	40.17	41.67	31.00	33.17	35.33	37.67	38.67	40.67
Set_2 (SL 1:2)	32.00	34.17	36.50	38.83	41.00	42.17	32.00	34.00	36.50	38.50	39.50	41.00
Set_3 (SL 1:3)	34.17	37.00	39.50	41.50	43.50	43.83	34.17	36.67	39.67	41.00	41.67	43.67
Set_4 (SL 2:1)	30.67	32.67	34.83	36.50	38.00	39.17	31.17	33.17	35.17	36.67	38.00	39.50
Set_5 (SL 3:1)	29.67	31.83	33.50	34.50	36.67	37.83	29.50	31.17	31.67	33.67	35.83	37.83
Average	31.57	33.80	36.10	37.97	39.87	40.93	31.57	33.63	35.67	37.50	38.73	40.53

CD at 5% = 0.50 at 1% = 0.66

Table 9.5 : The interaction effect of temperature, sources of milk, fat and starter culture on body and texture on score of yoghurt

Starter culture	Source of milk x Temperature x Fat											
	M₁ (cow milk)						M₂ (buffalo milk)					
	T₁ (39°C)			T₂ (42 °C)			T₁ (39 °C)			T₂ (42 °C)		
	F₁ (4%)	F₂ (5%)	F₃ (6%)	F₁ (4%)	F₂ (5%)	F₃ (6%)	F₁ (4%)	F₂ (5%)	F₃ (6%)	F₁ (4%)	F₂ (5%)	F₃ (6%)
Set₁ (SL 1:1)	24.30	24.43	24.55	24.57	24.90	25.10	24.47	24.73	24.93	24.83	25.13	25.43
Set₂ (SL 1:2)	24.53	24.60	24.73	24.67	25.03	25.37	24.58	24.87	25.15	25.00	25.37	25.63
Set₃ (SL 1:3)	25.17	25.63	25.90	25.48	25.93	26.33	25.43	25.90	26.17	25.90	26.50	26.93
Set₄ (SL 2:1)	24.07	24.50	24.03	24.60	24.80	25.03	24.60	24.77	25.00	24.67	25.10	25.33
Set₅ (SL 3:1)	23.89	24.43	23.70	24.43	24.67	24.73	24.40	24.67	24.83	24.57	24.87	25.17
Average	24.39	24.72	24.58	24.75	25.07	25.31	24.70	24.99	25.22	24.99	25.39	25.70

Not significant

Table 9.6 : The interaction effect of temperature, sources of milk, fat and starter culture on acidity on score of yoghurt

Starter culture	Source of milk x Temperature x Fat											
	M₁ (cow milk)						M₂ (buffalo milk)					
	T₁ (39°C)			T₂ (42 °C)			T₁ (39 °C)			T₂ (42 °C)		
	F₁ (4%)	F₂ (5%)	F₃ (6%)	F₁ (4%)	F₂ (5%)	F₃ (6%)	F₁ (4%)	F₂ (5%)	F₃ (6%)	F₁ (4%)	F₂ (5%)	F₃ (6%)
Set₁ (SL 1:1)	10.80	10.97	11.20	11.00	11.20	11.27	10.90	11.13	11.27	11.03	11.13	11.40
Set₂ (SL 1:2)	11.17	11.13	11.33	11.17	11.40	11.50	11.37	11.33	11.40	11.33	11.40	11.63
Set₃ (SL 1:3)	11.90	12.07	12.50	11.77	11.93	12.10	11.90	12.00	12.17	12.03	12.30	12.53
Set₄ (SL 2:1)	10.57	10.67	10.80	10.90	11.10	11.17	10.70	10.73	10.80	10.83	11.00	11.10
Set₅ (SL 3:1)	10.47	10.50	10.43	10.67	10.70	10.83	10.57	10.60	10.63	10.63	10.80	10.90
Average	10.98	11.07	11.25	11.10	11.27	11.37	11.09	11.16	11.25	11.17	11.33	11.51

Not significant

Table 9.7 : The interaction effect of temperature, sources of milk, fat and starter culture on colour and appearance on score of yoghurt

Starter culture	Source of milk x Temperature x Fat											
	M₁ (cow milk)						M₂ (buffalo milk)					
	T₁ (39°C)			T₂ (42 °C)			T₁ (39 °C)			T₂ (42 °C)		
	F_1 (4%)	F_2 (5%)	F_3 (6%)	F_1 (4%)	F_2 (5%)	F_3 (6%)	F_1 (4%)	F_2 (5%)	F_3 (6%)	F_1 (4%)	F_2 (5%)	F_3 (6%)
Set₁ (SL 1:1)	3.17	3.60	3.83	3.27	3.63	3.85	3.62	3.78	4.00	3.68	3.83	4.07
Set₂ (SL 1:2)	3.17	3.57	3.83	3.27	3.64	3.85	3.62	3.78	4.00	3.68	3.83	4.07
Set₃ (SL 1:3)	3.20	3.53	3.83	3.27	3.65	3.85	3.60	3.80	4.00	3.68	3.83	4.07
Set₄ (SL 2:1)	3.23	3.60	3.80	3.20	3.64	3.85	3.58	3.78	4.03	3.70	3.85	4.07
Set₅ (SL 3:1)	3.27	3.62	3.83	3.27	3.62	3.85	3.62	3.75	4.05	3.67	3.83	4.70
Average	3.21	3.58	3.83	3.25	3.63	3.85	3.61	3.78	4.02	3.68	3.84	4.70

Not significant

Table 9.8 : The interaction effect of temperature, sources of milk, SNF and starter culture on flavour on score of yoghurt

Starter culture	Source of milk x Temperature x SNF											
	M₁ (cow milk)						M₂ (buffalo milk)					
	T₁ (39°C)			T₂ (42 °C)			T₁ (39 °C)			T₂ (42 °C)		
	S_1 (10%)	S_2 (11%)	S_3 (12%)	S_1 (10%)	S_2 (11%)	S_3 (12%)	S_1 (10%)	S_2 (11%)	S_3 (12%)	S_1 (10%)	F2 (11%)	F3 (12%)
Set₁ (SL 1:1)	31.33	33.33	36.17	38.50	40.17	41.67	31.00	33.17	35.33	37.67	38.67	40.67
Set₂ (SL 1:2)	32.00	34.17	36.50	38.83	41.00	42.17	32.00	34.00	36.50	38.50	39.50	41.00
Set₃ (SL 1:3)	34.17	37.00	39.50	41.50	43.50	43.83	34.17	36.67	39.67	41.00	41.67	43.67
Set₄ (SL 2:1)	30.67	32.67	34.83	36.50	38.00	39.17	31.17	33.17	35.17	36.67	38.00	39.50
Set₅ (SL 3:1)	29.67	31.83	33.50	34.50	36.67	37.83	29.50	31.17	31.67	33.67	35.83	37.83
Average	31.57	33.80	36.10	37.97	39.87	40.93	31.57	33.63	35.67	37.50	38.73	40.53

Not significant

Table 9.9 : The interaction effect of temperature, sources of milk, SNF and starter culture on body and texture on score of yoghurt

Starter culture	Source of milk x Temperature x SNF											
	M₁ (cow milk)						M₂ (buffalo milk)					
	T₁ (39°C)			T₂ (42 °C)			T₁ (39 °C)			T₂ (42 °C)		
	S_1 (10%)	S_2 (11%)	S_3 (12%)	S_1 (10%)	S_2 (11%)	S_3 (12%)	S_1 (10%)	S_2 (11%)	S_3 (12%)	S_1 (10%)	F2 (11%)	F3 (12%)
Set₁ (SL 1:1)	32.67	33.67	34.50	39.67	40.00	40.67	32.50	33.17	33.83	38.30	39.00	39.67
Set₂ (SL 1:2)	33.33	34.17	35.17	40.33	40.50	41.17	33.50	34.17	34.83	39.17	39.67	40.17
Set₃ (SL 1:3)	36.00	36.83	37.83	42.83	42.67	43.33	36.17	36.67	37.67	41.67	41.83	42.83
Set₄ (SL 2:1)	32.00	32.67	33.50	37.50	37.83	38.33	32.50	33.00	34.00	37.50	37.83	38.83
Set₅ (SL 3:1)	31.00	31.67	32.33	35.67	36.17	37.17	30.33	30.67	31.33	35.00	35.67	36.67
Average	33.00	33.80	34.67	39.20	39.43	40.13	33.00	33.53	34.33	38.33	38.80	39.63

Not significant

Table 10.0 : The interaction effect of temperature, sources of milk, SNF and starter culture on body and texture on score of yoghurt

Starter culture	Source of milk x Temperature x SNF											
	M₁ (cow milk)						M₂ (buffalo milk)					
	T₁ (39°C)			T₂ (42 °C)			T₁ (39 °C)			T₂ (42 °C)		
	S_1 (10%)	S_2 (11%)	S_3 (12%)	S_1 (10%)	S_2 (11%)	S_3 (12%)	S_1 (10%)	S_2 (11%)	S_3 (12%)	S_1 (10%)	F2 (11%)	F3 (12%)
Set₁ (SL 1:1)	22.53	24.03	26.72	22.93	24.50	27.13	22.77	24.40	26.97	23.23	24.90	27.27
Set₂ (SL 1:2)	22.73	24.30	26.83	23.13	24.60	27.33	22.93	24.52	27.15	23.37	25.13	27.50
Set₃ (SL 1:3)	23.83	25.07	27.80	24.10	25.22	28.43	23.90	25.33	28.27	24.47	26.07	28.80
Set₄ (SL 2:1)	23.03	23.93	25.63	23.33	24.07	27.03	23.27	24.03	27.07	23.47	24.33	27.30
Set₅ (SL 3:1)	22.99	23.80	25.23	23.13	23.80	26.90	23.07	23.90	26.93	23.30	24.20	27.10
Average	23.03	24.23	26.44	23.33	24.44	27.37	23.19	24.44	27.28	23.57	24.93	27.59

Not significant

Table 10.1 : The interaction effect of temperature, sources of milk, and starter culture on acidity score of yoghurt

Starter culture	Source of milk x Temperature x SNF											
	M$_1$ (cow milk)						M$_2$ (buffalo milk)					
	T$_1$ (39°C)			T$_2$ (42 °C)			T$_1$ (39 °C)			T$_2$ (42 °C)		
	S$_1$ (10%)	S$_2$ (11%)	S$_3$ (12%)	S$_1$ (10%)	S$_2$ (11%)	S$_3$ (12%)	S$_1$ (10%)	S$_2$ (11%)	S$_3$ (12%)	S$_1$ (10%)	F2 (11%)	F3 (12%)
Set$_1$ (SL 1:1)	10.80	11.00	11.17	11.00	11.17	11.30	10.97	11.10	11.23	11.07	11.17	11.33
Set$_2$ (SL 1:2)	11.07	11.23	11.33	11.23	41.00	11.47	11.17	11.30	11.63	11.33	11.43	11.60
Set$_3$ (SL 1:3)	11.90	12.13	12.43	11.63	43.50	12.23	11.80	12.00	12.27	12.03	12.27	12.57
Set$_4$ (SL 2:1)	10.50	10.67	10.87	10.93	38.00	11.17	10.63	10.73	10.87	10.87	10.97	11.10
Set$_5$ (SL 3:1)	10.30	10.50	10.60	10.60	36.67	10.87	10.47	10.60	10.73	10.70	10.77	10.87
Average	10.91	11.11	11.28	11.08	39.87	11.41	11.01	11.15	11.35	11.20	11.32	11.49

Not significant

Table 10.2 : The interaction effect of temperature, sources of milk, SNF and starter culture on colour and appearance score of yoghurt

Starter culture	Source of milk x Temperature x SNF											
	M$_1$ (cow milk)						M$_2$ (buffalo milk)					
	T$_1$ (39°C)			T$_2$ (42 °C)			T$_1$ (39 °C)			T$_2$ (42 °C)		
	S$_1$ (10%)	S$_2$ (11%)	S$_3$ (12%)	S$_1$ (10%)	S$_2$ (11%)	S$_3$ (12%)	S$_1$ (10%)	S$_2$ (11%)	S$_3$ (12%)	S$_1$ (10%)	F2 (11%)	F3 (12%)
Set$_1$ (SL 1:1)	3.40	3.53	3.67	3.45	3.58	3.72	3.67	3.77	3.97	3.73	3.82	4.03
Set$_2$ (SL 1:2)	3.37	3.53	3.67	3.45	3.58	3.72	3.67	3.77	3.97	3.73	3.82	4.03
Set$_3$ (SL 1:3)	3.40	3.53	3.63	3.45	3.60	3.72	3.63	3.77	4.00	3.73	3.82	4.03
Set$_4$ (SL 2:1)	3.40	3.57	3.67	3.42	3.55	3.72	3.63	3.77	4.00	3.73	3.85	4.03
Set$_5$ (SL 3:1)	3.43	3.57	3.70	3.45	3.58	3.70	3.68	3.73	4.00	3.75	3.82	4.00
Average	3.40	3.55	3.67	3.45	3.58	3.71	3.66	3.76	3.99	3.74	3.82	4.03

Not significant

4.1.17 Interaction effect of temperature, sources of milks, fat and starter culture on physical attributes of yoghurt

Flavour

The data presented in table-9.5 clearly indicate that flavour of cow and buffalo milk yoghurt prepared at both temperature, increased significantly (P < 0.01) with increase in the concentration of fat in milk, irrespective of starter culture used. It was also observed that the flavour quality of yoghurt improved significantly (P < 0.01) due to combined effects of all the physical attributes on the samples. The highest flavour score (43.83) was recorded in interaction group $M_1 \times T_2 \times F_1 \times Set_5$.

The interaction effects of temperature, sources of milk, fat and starter culture on body & textural, acidity score and colour & appearance of yoghurt was statistically not significant (Table-9.6, 9.7 and 9.8).

Interaction effect of T x M x S x ST, T x F x S x ST, F x M x S x ST and T x M x F x S x ST on flavour, body & texture, acidity and colour & appearance score of yoghurt were statistically not significant (Table 9.9-11.4)

B. Chemical attributes

4.2 Effect of various factors on chemical attributes (fat, protein, lactose, ash, acidity and pH) of yoghurt

4.2.1 Source of milk

A perusal of data presented in the table (Table-11.5) clearly indicate that the per cent, fat protein, lactose, ash and acidity in yoghurt were 5.02, 4.72, 5.19, 1.02 and 0.97 in cow milk yoghurt and 5.02, 4.72, 5.32, 1.02 and 0.98 per cent in buffalo milk yoghurt, respectively. Cow and buffalo milk yoghurt did not differ with each other in the constituents of fat, protein and ash. The variations were observed only in lactose, acidity and pH value of yoghurt. The lactose and acidity values in buffalo milk yoghurt were significantly (P < 0.01) higher than the values observed in cow milk yoghurt whereas, buffalo milk yoghurt was significantly (P < 0.01) lower in respect of pH than the value observed in cow milk yoghurt.

By nature, buffalo milk contained more fat than cow milk. In the present experiment fat and SNF were adjusted by adding cream and skim milk powder at the same level in cow and buffalo milk both. Owing to this fat, protein and ash which are the main part of total solids did not differs in the yoghurt prepared from both the milk. The higher lactose, acidity and lower pH value in buffalo milk yoghurt may be due to the some basic compositional variations in cow and buffalo milk as they were not disturbed in the milk. Akin and Konar (1993) reported that type of milk had significant (P < 0.05) effect on pH, titrable acidity, fat protein and total sugar of yoghurt. Singh and Kaul (1982) observed that the cultures grown in buffalo milk produced more acidity than cultures grown in cow's and goat's milk. This result is parallel to the findings observed in the present experiment, where higher acidity and lactose and lower pH value were observed in buffalo milk yoghurt.

4.2.2 Temperature

The data presented in table-11.5 clearly show that the variation in incubation temperature did not affect the fat, protein and ash content of yogurt. The fat (5.02%), protein (4.72%) and ash content (1.02%) values recorded in yoghurt sample prepared at lower temperature (39°C) were the same as observed in the sample prepared at higher temperature (42°C). Yoghurt prepared at 39°C & 42°C incubation temperature contained 5.32 & 5.19% lactose and 0.96 & 1.00% lactic acid with pH value of 4.57 & 4.52, respectively. The pH value recorded in yoghurt prepared at lower temperature was significantly (P < 0.01) higher than the value recorded at higher temperature whereas the acidity value in yoghurt prepared at lower temperature was significantly (P < 0.01) lower than the value recorded at higher temperature.

The reduction in lactose content and pH value and increase in lactic acid content of yoghurt at higher temperature may be due to the favourable growth of bacteria which are directly responsible for conversion of lactose to lactic acid in the fermented milk products. Cho-Ah-Ying et al. (1990) were also in view that temperature significantly ($P < 0.01$) affect the acidity of yoghurt as found in the present case.

The interaction effects of temperature & sources of milk and temperature & fat on fat, protein, lactose, ash, acidity and pH of yoghurt were not significant (Table 11.6-12.7).

Table 11.6 : The interaction effect of temperature and sources of milk on fat content (%) of yoghurt

Sources of milk	Temperature	
	T_1 (39^{0}C)	T_2 (42^{0}C)
M_1 (Cow milk)	5.02	5.02
M_2 (Buffalo milk)	5.02	5.02
Average	5.02	5.02

Not significant

Table 11.7 : The interaction effect of temperature and sources of milk on protein content (%) of yoghurt

Not signification

Table 11.8 : The interaction effect of temperature and sources
of milk on lactose content (%) of yoghurt

Sources of milk	Temperature	
	T_1 (39^{0}C)	T_2 (42^{0}C)
M_1 (Cow milk)	5.23	5.14
M_2 (Buffalo milk)	5.40	5.24
Average	5.32	5.19

Not significant

Table 11.9 : The interaction effect of temperature and sources
of milk on ash content (%) of yoghurt

Sources of milk	Temperature	
	T_1 (39^{0}C)	T_2 (42^{0}C)
M_1 (Cow milk)	1.02	1.02
M_2 (Buffalo milk)	1.02	1.02
Average	1.02	1.02

Not significant

Table 12.0 : The interaction effect of temperature and sources
of milk on lactic acid content (%) of yoghurt

Sources of milk	Temperature	
	T_1 (39^{0}C)	T_2 (42^{0}C)
M_1 (Cow milk)	4.72	4.72
M_2 (Buffalo milk)	4.72	4.72
Average	4.72	4.72

Not significant

Table 12.1 : The interaction effect of temperature and sources
of milk on pH of yoghurt

Sources of milk	Temperature	
	T_1 (39^{0}C)	T_2 (42^{0}C)
M_1 (Cow milk)	4.58	4.53
M_2 (Buffalo milk)	4.57	4.52
Average	4.57	4.52

Not significant

Table 12.2 : The interaction effect of temperature and fat on fat content (%) of yoghurt

Temperature	Fat		
	F_1 (4%)	F_2 (5%)	F_3 (6%)
T_1 (39°C)	4.02	5.01	6.02
T_2 (42°C)	4.03	5.02	6.02
Average	4.02	5.02	6.02

Not significant

Table 12.3 : The interaction effect of temperature and fat on protein content (%) of yoghurt

Temperature	Fat		
	F_1 (4%)	F_2 (5%)	F_3 (6%)
T_1 (39°C)	4.72	4.72	4.72
T_2 (42°C)	4.71	4.72	4.72
Average	4.71	4.72	4.72

Not significant

Table 12.4 : The interaction effect of temperature and fat on lactose content (%) of yoghurt

Temperature	Fat		
	F_1 (4%)	F_2 (5%)	F_3 (6%)
T_1 (39°C)	5.34	5.34	5.28
T_2 (42°C)	5.18	5.23	5.17
Average	5.26	5.28	5.22

Not significant

Table 12.5 : The interaction effect of temperature and fat on ash content (%) of yoghurt

Temperature	Fat		
	F_1 (4%)	F_2 (5%)	F_3 (6%)
T_1 (39°C)	1.02	1.02	1.02
T_2 (42°C)	1.01	1.02	1.02
Average	1.02	1.02	1.02

Not significant

Table 12.6 : The interaction effect of temperature and fat on lactic acid (%) content of yoghurt

Temperature	Fat		
	F_1 (4%)	F_2 (5%)	F_3 (6%)
T_1 (39°C)	0.96	0.96	0.96
T_2 (42°C)	0.99	1.00	1.00
Average	0.98	0.98	0.98

Not significant

Table 12.7 : The interaction effect of temperature and fat on pH of yoghurt

Temperature	Fat		
	F_1 (4%)	F_2 (5%)	F_3 (6%)
T_1 (39°C)	4.58	4.57	4.56
T_2 (42°C)	4.53	4.52	4.52
Average	4.55	4.55	4.54

Not significant

4.2.2.1 Interaction effect of temperature and SNF on chemical attributes of yoghurt

Acidity

The data presented in table 13.2 depict that the acidity of yoghurt significantly ($P < 0.05$) increased as the concentration of SNF increases in the milk during preparation of yoghurt at both the temperature levels. The average acidity were noted as 0.91, 0.97, 1.00, 0.96, 1.00 and 1.03 per cent in interaction groups T_1S_1, T_1S_2, T_1S_3, T_2S_1, T_2S_2 and T_2S_3, respectively. The percentage acidity recorded in interaction groups T_2S_1, T_1S_2, T_1S_3, T_2S_1, T_2S2 and T_2S_3 were comparatively higher ($P < 0.05$) than the acidity recorded in interaction groups T_1S_1, T_1S_2 and T_1S_3. It was also noted that the acidity recorded in interaction groups T_1S_1, T_1S_2 and T_1S_3. It was also noted that the lactic acid content in yoghurt samples were increased significantly ($P < 0.05$) when incubation temperature increased from 39°C to

42°C, irrespective of the levels of SNF included in the milk. The highest acidity percentage (1.03%) was recorded in interaction groups T_2S_3 and the lowest (0.91%) was observed in interaction group T_1S_1.

pH

The pH value of yoghurt samples reduced significantly (P < 0.01) as the level of temperature enhanced from 39°C to 42°C, irrespective of the amount of SNF added in the milk (Table-13.3). The average pH value were noted as 4.65, 4.55, 4.53, 4.55, 4.52 and 4.49 in interaction groups T1S1, T1S2, T1S3, T_2S_1, T_2S_2 and T_2S_3 respectively. The pH of yoghurt was also reduced significantly (P < 0.01) at every increase in SNF level of milk, irrespective of incubation temperature. The pH value recorded in yoghurt samples prepared at 420C in association with different levels of SNF in milk were significantly (P < 0.01) lower than the pH value recorded in the samples prepared at 390C. The highest pH value (4.65) was noted in yoghurt sample prepared at lower temperature in association with lower level of SNF in milk, whereas, the lowest value (4.51) was observed in the sample prepared at higher temperature in combination with the highest level of SNF in milk.

The interaction effects of temperature and SNF on other chemical attributes viz; fat, protein, lactose and ash were not significant (Table – 12.8, 12.9, 13.0 and 13.1).

Table 12.8 : The interaction effect of temperature and SNF on fat content (%) of yoghurt

Temperature	SNF		
	S_1 (10%)	S_2 (11%)	S_3 (12%)
T_1 (39°C)	5.02	5.02	5.01
T_2 (42°C)	5.02	5.03	5.02
Average	5.02	5.03	5.02

Not significant

Table 12.9 : The interaction effect of temperature and SNF on protein content (%) of yoghurt

Temperature	SNF		
	S_1 (10%)	S_2 (11%)	S_3 (12%)
T_1 (39°C)	4.29	4.67	5.19
T_2 (42°C)	4.29	4.67	5.19
Average	4.29	4.67	5.19

Not significant

Table 13.0 : The interaction effect of temperature and SNF on lactose content (%) of yoghurt

Temperature	SNF		
	S_1 (10%)	S_2 (11%)	S_3 (12%)
T_1 (39°C)	4.88	5.30	5.77
T_2 (42°C)	4.74	5.20	5.63
Average	4.81	5.25	5.70

Not significant

Table 13.1 : The interaction effect of temperature and SNF on ash content (%) of yoghurt

Temperature	SNF		
	S_1 (10%)	S_2 (11%)	S_3 (12%)
T_1 (39°C)	0.88	0.97	1.20
T_2 (42°C)	0.88	0.97	1.20
Average	0.88	0.97	1.20

Not significant

Table 13.2 : The interaction effect of temperature and SNF on lactic acid (%) content of yoghurt

Temperature	SNF		
	S_1 (10%)	S_2 (11%)	S_3 (12%)
T_1 (39°C)	0.91	0.97	1.00
T_2 (42°C)	0.96	1.00	1.03
Average	0.94	0.98	1.01

CD at 5% = 0.006, at 1% = NS

Table 13.3 : The interaction effect of temperature and SNF on pH of yoghurt

Temperature	SNF		
	S_1 (10%)	S_2 (11%)	S_3 (12%)
T_1 (39°C)	4.65	4.55	4.53
T_2 (42°C)	4.55	4.52	4.49
Average	4.60	4.53	4.51

CD at 5% = 0.02 at 1% = 0.015

4.2.2.2 Interaction effect of temperature and starter culture on chemical attributes of yoghurt

Acidity

It can be seen from the table (Table-13.8) that the observed values in respect of acidity in yoghurt samples were 0.88, (T1 Set1), 0.89% (T_1 Set$_2$), 0.09% (T_1Set$_3$), 1.06% (T_1 Set$_4$), 1.08% (T_1 Set$_5$), 0.90% (T_2 Set$_1$), 0.09% (T_2 Set$_2$), 0.94% (T_2 Set$_3$), 1.90% (T_2 Set$_4$), 1.14 % (T_2 Set$_5$). At all temperature levels, the lactic acid content of yoghurt increased significantly (P < 0.01) as the proportion of lactobacilli and streptococci increases in the culture. Further, it was also noted that acidity observed in the samples prepared at 42°C with various proportions of lactobacilli and streptococci in the culture were significant (P <0.01) higher than the acidity recored in samples prepared at lower temperature (39°C).The sample prepared at 42°C in association with SL 3:1 culture group had the maximum (1.4%) acidity content whereas, the sample prepared at lower temperature in combination with SL 1:1 culture groups recorded the least acidity (0.88%).

pH

The pH value of yoghurt significantly (P < 0.01) reduced as the concentration of lactobacilli and streptococci increases in the culturel, irrespective of incubation temperature (Table-13.9) used. The pH values were noted as 4.67, 4.63, 4.61,4.49, 4.46, 4.60, 4.58, 4.56, and 4.41 in interaction groups T_1 Set$_1$, and T_1 Set$_2$, T_1 Set$_3$,T_1 Set$_4$, T_1 Set$_5$, T_2 Set$_1$, T_2 Set$_2$, T_2 Set$_3$, T_2 Set$_4$, and T_2 Set$_5$, respectively. The yoghurt samples prepared at 420C with different proportions of lactobacilli and streptococci in the culture had lower pH value than the samples prepared at lower temperature (39°C). The maximum pH value. 4.67 was recorded in sample prepared at lower temperature in combination with Set$_1$ culture group and the lowest value (4.44) was recorded in sample prepared at higher temperature in association with group SL 3:1.

Table 13.4 : The interaction effect of temperature and starter culture on fat content (%) of yoghurt

Temperature	Starter Culture				
	Set$_1$ (SL 1:1)	Set$_2$ (SL 1:2)	Set$_3$ (SL 1:3)	Set$_4$ (SL 2:1)	Set$_5$ (SL 3:1)
T_1 (39 °C)	5.03	5.01	5.02	5.03	5.01
T_2 (42 °C)	5.03	5.01	5.02	5.03	5.02
Average	5.03	5.01	5.02	5.03	5.01

Not significant

Table 13.5 : The interaction effect of temperature and starter culture on protein content (%) of yoghurt

Temperature	Starter Culture				
	Set$_1$ (SL 1:1)	Set$_2$ (SL 1:2)	Set$_3$ (SL 1:3)	Set$_4$ (SL 2:1)	Set$_5$ (SL 3:1)
T_1 (39 °C)	4.71	4.73	4.71	4.72	4.72
T_2 (42 °C)	4.71	4.73	4.71	4.72	4.72
Average	4.71	4.73	4.71	4.72	4.72

Not significant

Table 13.6 : The interaction effect of temperature and starter culture on lactose content (%) of yoghurt

Temperature	Starter Culture				
	Set$_1$ (SL 1:1)	Set$_2$ (SL 1:2)	Set$_3$ (SL 1:3)	Set$_4$ (SL 2:1)	Set$_5$ (SL 3:1)
T_1 (39 °C)	5.27	5.45	5.60	5.21	5.06
T_2 (42 °C)	5.11	5.32	5.51	5.06	5.96
Average	5.19	5.38	5.56	5.13	5.01

Not significant

Table 13.7 : The interaction effect of temperature and starter culture on ash content (%) of yoghurt

Temperature	Starter Culture				
	Set_1 (SL 1:1)	Set_2 (SL 1:2)	Set_3 (SL 1:3)	Set_4 (SL 2:1)	Set_5 (SL 3:1)
T_1 (39 ^{0}C)	1.01	1.01	1.01	1.03	1.03
T_2 (42 ^{0}C)	1.01	1.01	1.01	1.03	1.05
Average	1.01	1.01	1.01	1.03	1.02

Not significant

Table 13.8 : The interaction effect of temperature and starter culture on lactic acid content (%) of yoghurt

Temperature	Starter Culture				
	Set_1 (SL 1:1)	Set_2 (SL 1:2)	Set_3 (SL 1:3)	Set_4 (SL 2:1)	Set_5 (SL 3:1)
T_1 (39 ^{0}C)	0.88	0.89	0.90	1.06	1.08
T_2 (42 ^{0}C)	0.90	0.91	0.94	1.09	1.14
Average	0.89	0.90	0.92	1.08	1.11

CD at 5% = 0.008 at 1% = 0.011

Table 13.9 : The interaction effect of temperature and starter culture on pH of yoghurt

Temperature	Starter Culture				
	Set_1 (SL 1:1)	Set_2 (SL 1:2)	Set_3 (SL 1:3)	Set_4 (SL 2:1)	Set_5 (SL 3:1)
T_1 (39 ^{0}C)	4.67	4.63	4.61	4.49	4.46
T_2 (42 ^{0}C)	4.60	4.58	4.56	4.46	4.41
Average	4.63	4.61	4.59	4.47	4.44

CD at 5% = 0.015 at 1% = 0.020

4.2.3 Fat

It is clear from the data presented in table-11.5 that the average fat content in yoghurt increased ($P < 0.01$) as the levels of fat increases in the milk but, the other chemical constituents (protein, lactose, ash and acidity of yoghurt) did not differ significantly on increase or decrease in the levels of milk fat.

The pH value of yoghurt significantly (P < 0.05) decreased when fat content in milk increased from 5.0 to 6.0 per cent. The values for fat, protein, lactose, ash, lactic acid and pH were 4.02%, 4.71%, 5.26%, 1.02%, 4.72%, 5.28%, 1.02%, 0.98 and 4.55 in the sample prepared with 5.0% fat and 6.02%, 4.72%, 5.22%, 1.02%, 0.98% and 4.54% in the sample prepared with 5.0% fat and 6.02%, 4.72%, 5.22%, 1.02%, 0.98% and 4.54% in the sample prepared from the milk containing 6.0% fat.

Dolezak and Vokacova (1981) found that the acidity of yoghurt apparently increased as the fat content in milk increases. This result is not corroborate with the result observed in present study.

4.2.3.1 Interaction effect of fat & sources of milk, fat & SNF and fat & starter culture of chemical attributes of yoghurt

The fat & sources of milk, fat & SNF and fat & starter culture had no any significant interaction impact on chemical attributes of yoghurt. The statistically analysed data are presented in the table (Table 14.0 to 15.7).

Table 14.0 : The interaction effect of fat and sources of milk on fat content (%) of yoghurt

Sources of milk	Fat		
	F_1 (4%)	F_2 (5%)	F_3 (6%)
M_1 (Cow milk)	4.03	5.02	6.02
M_2 (Buffalo milk)	4.02	5.02	6.02
Average	4.02	5.02	6.02

Not significant

Table 14.1 : The interaction effect of fat and sources of milk on protein content (%) of yoghurt

Sources of milk	Fat		
	F_1 (4%)	F_2 (5%)	F_3 (6%)
M_1 (Cow milk)	4.71	4.72	4.72
M_2 (Buffalo milk)	4.72	4.72	4.72
Average	4.71	4.72	4.72

Not significant

Table 14.2 : The interaction effect of fat and sources of milk on lactose content (%) of yoghurt

Sources of milk	Fat		
	F_1 (4%)	F_2 (5%)	F_3 (6%)
M_1 (Cow milk)	5.19	5.21	5.17
M_2 (Buffalo milk)	5.33	5.36	5.27
Average	5.26	5.28	5.22

Not significant

Table 14.3 : The interaction effect of fat and sources of milk on ash content (%) of yoghurt

Sources of milk	Fat		
	F_1 (4%)	F_2 (5%)	F_3 (6%)
M_1 (Cow milk)	1.02	1.02	1.02
M_2 (Buffalo milk)	1.02	1.02	1.02
Average	1.02	1.02	1.02

Not significant

Table 14.4 : The interaction effect of fat and sources of milk on lactic acid content (%) of yoghurt

Sources of milk	Fat		
	F_1 (4%)	F_2 (5%)	F_3 (6%)
M_1 (Cow milk)	0.97	0.97	0.98
M_2 (Buffalo milk)	0.98	0.98	0.98
Average	0.98	0.98	0.98

Not significant

Table 14.5 : The interaction effect of fat and sources of milk on pH of yoghurt

Sources of milk	Fat		
	F_1 (4%)	F_2 (5%)	F_3 (6%)
M_1 (Cow milk)	4.56	4.55	4.55
M_2 (Buffalo milk)	4.55	4.54	4.54
Average	4.55	4.55	4.54

Not significant

Table 14.6 : The interaction of fat and SNF of fat content (%)
          of yoghurt

Fat	SNF		
	S_1 (10%)	S_2 (11%)	S_3 (12%)
F_1 (4%)	4.02	4.04	4.02
F_2 (5%)	5.02	5.00	5.02
F_3 (6%)	6.01	6.04	6.01
Average	5.02	5.03	5.02

Not significant

Table 14.7 : The interaction effect of fat and SNF on protein
          content (%) of yoghurt

Fat	SNF		
	S_1 (10%)	S_2 (11%)	S_3 (12%)
F_1 (4%)	4.29	4.66	5.19
F_2 (5%)	4.29	4.68	5.19
F_3 (6%)	4.29	4.67	5.19
Average	4.29	4.67	5.19

Not significant

Table 14.8 : The interaction effect of fat and SNF on lactose
          content (%) of yoghurt

Fat	SNF		
	S_1 (10%)	S_2 (11%)	S_3 (12%)
F_1 (4%)	4.83	4.66	5.19
F_2 (5%)	4.85	4.68	5.19
F_3 (6%)	4.74	4.67	5.19
Average	4.81	4.67	5.19

Not significant

Table 14.9 : The interaction effect of fat and SNF on ash content (%) of yoghurt

Fat	SNF		
	S_1 (10%)	S_2 (11%)	S_3 (12%)
F_1 (4%)	0.88	0.97	1.20
F_2 (5%)	0.88	0.97	1.21
F_3 (6%)	0.88	0.97	1.20
Average	0.88	0.97	1.20

Not significant

Table 15.0 : The interaction effect of fat and SNF on lactic acid content (%) of yoghurt

Fat	SNF		
	S_1 (10%)	S_2 (11%)	S_3 (12%)
F_1 (4%)	0.94	0.98	1.01
F_2 (5%)	0.94	0.98	1.01
F_3 (6%)	0.94	0.99	1.02
Average	0.94	0.98	1.01

Not significant

Table 15.1 : The interaction effect of fat and SNF on pH of yoghurt

Fat	SNF		
	S_1 (10%)	S_2 (11%)	S_3 (12%)
F_1 (4%)	4.61	4.54	4.52
F_2 (5%)	4.60	4.54	4.51
F_3 (6%)	4.59	4.53	4.50
Average	4.60	4.53	4.51

Not significant

Table 15.2 : The interaction effect of fat and starter culture on
          fat content (%) of yoghurt

Starter Culture	Fat		
	F_1 (4%)	F_2 (5%)	F_3 (6%)
Set1 (SL 1:1)	4.06	5.01	6.02
Set2 (SL 1:2)	4.01	5.00	6.02
Set3 (SL 1:3)	4.02	5.01	6.03
Set4 (SL 2:1)	4.04	5.03	6.02
Set5 (SL 3:1)	4.01	5.03	6.00
Average	4.02	5.02	6.02

Not significant

Table 15.3 : The interaction effect of fat and starter culture on
          protein content (%) of yoghurt

Starter Culture	Fat		
	F_1 (4%)	F_2 (5%)	F_3 (6%)
Set1 (SL 1:1)	5.19	5.21	5.18
Set2 (SL 1:2)	5.39	5.41	5.35
Set3 (SL 1:3)	5.58	5.58	5.50
Set4 (SL 2:1)	5.13	5.17	5.10
Set5 (SL 3:1)	5.00	5.05	4.98
Average	5.26	5.28	5.22

Not significant

Table 15.5 : The interaction effect of fat and starter culture on
          ash content (%) of yoghurt

Starter Culture	Fat		
	F_1 (4%)	F_2 (5%)	F_3 (6%)
Set1 (SL 1:1)	1.01	1.01	1.01
Set2 (SL 1:2)	1.01	1.01	1.01
Set3 (SL 1:3)	1.01	1.01	1.01
Set4 (SL 2:1)	1.03	1.03	1.03
Set5 (SL 3:1)	1.03	1.03	1.02
Average	1.02	1.02	1.02

Not significant

Table 15.6 : The interaction effect of fat and starter culture on lactic acid content (%) of yoghurt

Starter Culture	Fat		
	F_1 (4%)	F_2 (5%)	F_3 (6%)
Set1 (SL 1:1)	0.89	0.89	0.89
Set2 (SL 1:2)	0.90	0.90	0.90
Set3 (SL 1:3)	0.92	0.92	0.92
Set4 (SL 2:1)	1.07	1.08	1.08
Set5 (SL 3:1)	1.11	1.11	1.11
Average	0.98	0.98	0.98

Not significant

Table 15.7 : The interaction effect of fat and starter culture on pH of yoghurt

Starter Culture	Fat		
	F_1 (4%)	F_2 (5%)	F_3 (6%)
Set1 (SL 1:1)	4.64	4.63	4.63
Set2 (SL 1:2)	4.62	4.60	4.60
Set3 (SL 1:3)	4.59	4.59	4.58
Set4 (SL 2:1)	4.49	4.47	4.46
Set5 (SL 3:1)	4.44	4.44	4.43
Average	4.55	4.55	4.54

Not significant

4.2.4 SNF

The protein content in yoghurt significantly ($P < 0.01$) increased from 4.29% to 5.19% as the concentration of SNF increases from 10% to 12% in the milk (Table-11.5). Similarly, the lactose, ash, acidity content of yoghurt also increased significantly ($P < 0.01$) from 4.81% to 5.70%, 0.88% to 1.20% and 0.94% ot 1.01% respectively as the concentration of SNF increases from 10% to 12% in the milk. These values are inversely proportioned ($P < 0.01$) to the value of pH recored from the yoghurt sample. The levels of SNF had no any effect on the concentration of fat in yoghurt.

The increase in the protein, lactose and ash content of yoghurt might be due to increase in the levels of SNF in milk as it is positively correlated with the above milk constituents. The increase in acidity and decrease in pH value of yoghurt prepared from increasing levels of SNF in milk may be due to the increase in the protein, phosphate, citrate, lactates and other miscellaneous milk constituents in milk. Similar views have also been observed by Jennes and Patton (1959), Humphreys and Planket (1969) and Tamime et al. (1987) who found that the titrable acidity increased as the total solids content in milk increases.

4.2.4.1 Interaction effect of SNF and sources of milk on chemical attributes of yoghurt

The interaction effect of SNF and sources of milk on the chemical attribute of yoghurt have been presented in the table (Table-15.8 to 16.3) The values recorded from these table did not show any differences among the chemical attributes of yoghurt.

Table 15.8 : The interaction effect of SNF and sources of milk on fat content (%) of yoghurt

Sources of milk	SNF		
	S_1 (10%)	S_2 (11%)	S_3 (12%)
M_1 (Cow milk)	5.02	5.03	5.02
M_2 (Buffalo milk)	5.02	5.02	5.02
Average	5.02	5.03	5.02

Not significant

Table 15.9 : The interaction effect of SNF and sources of milk on protein content (%) of yoghurt

Sources of milk	SNF		
	S_1 (10%)	S_2 (11%)	S_3 (12%)
M_1 (Cow milk)	4.29	4.67	5.19
M_2 (Buffalo milk)	4.29	4.67	5.19
Average	4.29	4.67	5.19

Not significant

Table 16.0 : The interaction effect of SNF and sources of milk on lactose content (%) of yoghurt

Sources of milk	SNF		
	S_1 (10%)	S_2 (11%)	S_3 (12%)
M_1 (Cow milk)	4.74	5.19	5.64
M_2 (Buffalo milk)	4.88	5.32	5.77
Average	4.81	5.25	5.70

Not significant

Table 16.1 : The interaction effect of SNF and sources of milk on ash content (%) of yoghurt

Sources of milk	SNF		
	S_1 (10%)	S_2 (11%)	S_3 (12%)
M_1 (Cow milk)	0.88	0.97	1.20
M_2 (Buffalo milk)	0.88	0.97	1.20
Average	0.88	0.97	1.20

Not significant

Table 16.2 : The interaction effect of SNF and sources of milk on lactose content (%) of yoghurt

Sources of milk	SNF		
	S_1 (10%)	S_2 (11%)	S_3 (12%)
M_1 (Cow milk)	0.94	0.98	1.01
M_2 (Buffalo milk)	0.94	0.99	1.02
Average	0.94	0.98	1.01

Not significant

Table 16.3 : The interaction effect of SNF and sources of milk on pH of yoghurt

Sources of milk	SNF		
	S_1 (10%)	S_2 (11%)	S_3 (12%)
M_1 (Cow milk)	4.60	4.54	4.51
M_2 (Buffalo milk)	4.60	4.53	4.51
Average	4.60	4.53	4.51

Not significant

4.2.4.2 Interaction effects of SNF and starter culture on chemical attributes of yoghurt

Lactose

The observed values (Table-16.6) in respect to lactose content of yoghurt were 4.79% (Set$_1$ S$_1$), 5.13% (Set$_1$ S$_2$), 5.65% (Set$_1$ S$_3$), 4.91% (Set$_2$ S$_1$), 5.44% (Set$_2$ S$_2$), 5.92% (Set$_2$ S$_3$), 5.07% (Set$_3$ S$_1$). 5.55% (Set$_3$ S$_2$), 6.05% (Set$_3$ S$_3$), 4.69% (Set$_4$ S$_1$), 5.21% (Set$_4$ S$_2$), 5.50% (Set$_4$ S$_3$), 4.58% (Set$_5$ S$_1$), 5.06% (Set$_5$ S$_2$), and 5.39% (Set$_5$ S3). These values clearly indicate that the lactose content of yoghurt significantly (P < 0.01) increased as the concentraction of SNF increases in the milk, irrespective to starter culture used. The samples inoculated with SL 1:3 culture group had significantly (P <0.01) higher lactose content that the yoghurt obtained with culture groups SL 1:1, SL 1:2, SL 2:1, and SL 3:1, at all the levels of SNF. The maximum (6.05%) lactose percent was recorded in interaction group S3 x Set3 and the minimum (4.58%) value was observed in interaction group S$_1$ x Set$_5$.

Acidity

On increasing levels of SNF in milk, the acidity of yoghurt increased significantly (P < 0.01), irrespective of the starter culture used (Table 16.8). The acidity of yoghurt was also increased significantly (P < 0.01) as the concentration of lactobacilli and streptococci increases in the milk containing 10%, 11% and 12% SNF. The highest acidity (1.14%) was recorded in interaction group Set$_5$ x S$_3$ and the lowest value (0.86%) was observed in interaction group Set$_1$ x S$_1$.

pH

The pH values were noted as 4.71, 4.62, 4.57, 4.66, 4.60, 4.56, 4.63, 4.58, 4.55, 4.53, 4.45, 4.45, 4.48. 4.43 and 4.41 in interaction groups Set$_1$ S$_1$, Set$_1$ Set$_2$, Set$_1$ S$_3$, Set$_2$ S$_1$, Set$_2$ S$_2$, Set$_2$ S$_3$, Set$_3$ S$_1$, Set$_3$ S$_2$, Set$_3$ S$_3$, Set$_4$ S$_1$, Set$_4$ S$_2$, Set$_4$ S$_3$, Set$_5$ S$_1$, Set$_5$ S$_2$ and Set$_5$ S$_3$, respectively (Table 16.9). The pH of yoghurt reduced significantly (P < 0.01) as the levels of SNF increases in the milk, except interaction group $Set_4 S_3$ at all the levels of culture used. The pH of yoghurt was also reduced significantly (P < 0.01) as the proportion of lactobacilli increases in the milk containing 10.0% and 11.0% SNF. Further, it was also observed that the pH value decreased as the concentration of streptococci increases in the milk containing all the levels of SNF present in the milk.

The interaction effects of SNF and starter culture on fat, protein and ash content of yoghurt were statistically not significant (Table 16.4, 16.5 and 16.7).

Table 16.4 : The interaction effect of SNF and starter culture on fat content (%) of yoghurt

Starter culture	SNF		
	S_1 (10%)	S_2 (11%)	S_3 (12%)
Set_1 (SL 1:1)	5.03	5.03	5.03
Set_2 (SL 1:2)	5.01	5.01	5.01
Set_3 (SL 1:3)	5.02	5.03	5.01
Set_4 (SL 2:1)	5.02	5.04	5.03
Set_5 (SL 3:1)	5.02	5.01	5.01
Average	5.02	5.03	5.02

Not significant

Table 16.5 : The interaction effect of SNF and starter culture on lactose content (%) of yoghurt

Starter culture	SNF		
	S_1 (10%)	S_2 (11%)	S_3 (12%)
Set_1 (SL 1:1)	4.03	4.65	5.18
Set_2 (SL 1:2)	4.28	4.70	5.20
Set_3 (SL 1:3)	4.30	4.64	5.19
Set_4 (SL 2:1)	4.29	4.67	5.20
Set_5 (SL 3:1)	4.29	4.69	5.18
Average	4.29	4.67	5.19

Not significant

Table 16.6 : The interaction effect of SNF and starter culture
           on lactose content (%) of yoghurt

Starter culture	SNF		
	S_1 (10%)	S_2 (11%)	S_3 (12%)
Set$_1$ (SL 1:1)	4.79	5.13	5.65
Set$_2$ (SL 1:2)	4.91	5.33	5.92
Set$_3$ (SL 1:3)	5.07	5.55	6.05
Set$_4$ (SL 2:1)	4.69	5.21	5.50
Set$_5$ (SL 3:1)	4.58	5.06	5.39
Average	4.81	5.25	5.70

CD at 5% = 0.118 at 1% = 0.155

Table 16.7 : The interaction effect of SNF and starter culture
           on ash content (%) of yoghurt

Starter culture	SNF		
	S_1 (10%)	S_2 (11%)	S_3 (12%)
Set$_1$ (SL 1:1)	0.87	0.97	1.19
Set$_2$ (SL 1:2)	0.88	0.97	1.19
Set$_3$ (SL 1:3)	0.87	0.97	1.19
Set$_4$ (SL 2:1)	0.88	0.97	1.22
Set$_5$ (SL 3:1)	0.89	0.98	1.21
Average	0.88	0.97	1.20

Not significant

Table 16.8 : The interaction effect of SNF and starter culture
           on lactic acid content (%) of yoghurt

Starter culture	SNF		
	S_1 (10%)	S_2 (11%)	S_3 (12%)
Set$_1$ (SL 1:1)	0.86	0.88	0.92
Set$_2$ (SL 1:2)	0.87	0.89	0.94
Set$_3$ (SL 1:3)	0.87	0.93	0.95
Set$_4$ (SL 2:1)	1.01	1.10	1.12
Set$_5$ (SL 3:1)	1.07	1.12	1.14
Average	0.94	0.98	1.01

CD at 5% = 0.010 at 1% = 0.013

Table 16.9 : The interaction effect of SNF and starter culture on pH of yoghurt

Starter culture	SNF		
	S_1 (10%)	S_2 (11%)	S_3 (12%)
Set_1 (SL 1:1)	4.71	4.62	4.57
Set_2 (SL 1:2)	4.66	4.60	4.56
Set_3 (SL 1:3)	4.63	4.58	4.55
Set_4 (SL 2:1)	4.53	4.45	4.45
Set_5 (SL 3:1)	4.48	4.43	4.41
Average	4.60	4.53	4.51

CD at 5% = 0.019 at 1% = 0.024

4.2.5 Starter Culture

A least variation was observed in fat, protein and ash content of yoghurt sample prepared from any levels of bacterial inoculation in the milk (Table 11.5). The average lactose content in yoghurt was 5.19, 5.38, 5.56, 5.13 and 5.01 per cent when the sample inoculated with culture groups Set_1, Set_2, Set_3, Set_4 and Set_5 respectively. Samples contained 0.89, 0.90, 0.92, 1.08 and 1.11 per cent acidity whereas, pH values of yoghurt were recorded as 4.63, 4.61, 4.59, 4.47 and 4.44 in culture groups Set_1, Set_2, Set_3, Set_4 and Set_5 respectively. The lowest lactose content was noted in yoghurt prepared with culture group SL 3:1. Whereas the highest Value was observed in sample cogulated with SL 1:3. The lactic acid content in yoghurt significantly (P< 0.01) increased as the proportions of lactobacilli and streptococci increases in the culture. The sample fermented with SL 1:1 culture group had significantly (P <0.01) higher pH value than the value recorded from the samples fermented with culture groups SL 1:2, SL 1:3, SL 2:1 and SL 3:1.

The higher acidity content and lower pH value in yoghurt samples coagulated with culture group SL 3:1 may be due to the higher lactic acid produced by the streptococci bacteria in the product.

Kilic (1986) made yoghurt form cow milk by using culture of *S. thermophillus* and *L. bulgaricus* in the ratios of 1:1 and 0.8 : 1.2. He reported than the acidity of yoghurt varied accordingly to the cultures used as the result found in the present case.

The interaction effects of ST x M, T x M x F, T x M x S, T x M x ST, T x F x S and T x F x ST on all chemical attributes of yoghurt also were not statistically significantly (Table 17.0-20.5).

Table 17.0 : The interaction effect of starter culture and sources of milk on fat (%) content of yoghurt

Sources of milk	Starter culture				
	Set$_1$ (SL 1:1)	Set$_2$ (SL 1:2)	Set$_3$ (SL 1:3)	Set$_4$ (SL 2:1)	Set$_5$ (SL 3:1)
M$_1$ (Cow milk)	5.04	5.01	5.02	5.03	5.01
M$_2$ (Buffalo milk)	5.02	5.01	5.02	5.03	5.01
Average	5.03	5.01	5.02	5.03	5.01

Not significant

Table 17.1 : The interaction effect of starter culture and sources of milk on protein (%) content of yoghurt

Sources of milk	Starter culture				
	Set$_1$ (SL 1:1)	Set$_2$ (SL 1:2)	Set$_3$ (SL 1:3)	Set$_4$ (SL 2:1)	Set$_5$ (SL 3:1)
M$_1$ (Cow milk)	5.04	4.73	4.72	4.72	4.72
M$_2$ (Buffalo milk)	5.02	4.73	4.71	4.72	4.72
Average	5.03	4.73	4.71	4.72	7.72

Not significant

Table 17.2 : The interaction effect of starter culture and sources of milk on lactic acid content (%) of yoghurt

Sources of milk	Starter culture				
	Set$_1$ (SL 1:1)	Set$_2$ (SL 1:2)	Set$_3$ (SL 1:3)	Set$_4$ (SL 2:1)	Set$_5$ (SL 3:1)
M$_1$ (Cow milk)	5.12	5.32	5.48	5.07	4.95
M$_2$ (Buffalo milk)	5.26	5.45	5.63	5.20	5.07
Average	5.19	5.38	5.56	5.13	5.01

Not significant

Table 17.3 : The interaction effect of starter culture and sources of milk on ash content (%) of yoghurt

Sources of milk	Starter culture				
	Set₁ (SL 1:1)	Set₂ (SL 1:2)	Set₃ (SL 1:3)	Set₄ (SL 2:1)	Set₅ (SL 3:1)
M₁ (Cow milk)	1.01	1.01	1.01	1.03	1.03
M₂ (Buffalo milk)	1.01	1.01	1.01	1.03	1.02
Average	1.01	1.01	1.01	1.03	1.02

Not significant

Table 17.4 : The interaction effect of starter culture and sources of milk on lactic acid content (%) of yoghurt

Sources of milk	Starter culture				
	Set₁ (SL 1:1)	Set₂ (SL 1:2)	Set₃ (SL 1:3)	Set₄ (SL 2:1)	Set₅ (SL 3:1)
M₁ (Cow milk)	0.88	0.90	0.91	1.07	1.11
M₂ (Buffalo milk)	0.89	0.90	0.92	1.08	1.11
Average	0.89	0.90	0.92	1.08	1.11

Not significant

Table 17.5 : The interaction effect of starter culture and sources of milk on pH of yoghurt

Sources of milk	Starter culture				
	Set₁ (SL 1:1)	Set₂ (SL 1:2)	Set₃ (SL 1:3)	Set₄ (SL 2:1)	Set₅ (SL 3:1)
M₁ (Cow milk)	4.64	4.61	4.59	4.48	4.44
M₂ (Buffalo milk)	4.63	4.60	4.58	4.47	4.43
Average	4.63	4.61	4.59	4.47	4.44

Not significant

Table 17.6 : The interaction effect of temperature, sources of milk and fat on fat content (%) of yoghurt

Fat	Temperature x Sources of milk			
	M_1 (Cow milk)		M_2 (Buffalo milk)	
	T_1 (39%)	T_2 (42%)	T_1 (39%)	T_2 (42%)
F_1 (4%)	4.03	4.03	4.02	4.02
F_2 (5%)	5.01	5.02	5.02	5.02
F_3 (6%)	6.02	6.02	6.02	6.02
Average	5.02	5.02	5.02	5.02

Not significant

Table 17.7 : The interaction effect of temperature, sources of milk and fat on protein content (%) of yoghurt

Fat	Temperature x Sources of milk			
	M_1 (Cow milk)		M_2 (Buffalo milk)	
	T_1 (39%)	T_2 (42%)	T_1 (39%)	T_2 (42%)
F_1 (4%)	4.71	4.71	4.72	4.72
F_2 (5%)	4.72	4.71	4.72	4.72
F_3 (6%)	4.72	4.72	4.71	4.72
Average	4.72	4.72	4.72	4.72

Not significant

Table 17.8 : The interaction effect of temperature, sources of milk and fat on lactose content (%) of yoghurt

Fat	Temperature x Sources of milk			
	M_1 (Cow milk)		M_2 (Buffalo milk)	
	T_1 (39%)	T_2 (42%)	T_1 (39%)	T_2 (42%)
F_1 (4%)	5.24	5.13	5.43	5.23
F_2 (5%)	5.24	5.18	5.44	5.28
F_3 (6%)	5.22	5.12	5.33	5.21
Average	5.23	5.14	5.40	5.24

Not significant

Table 17.9 : The interaction effect of temperature, sources of milk and fat on ash content (%) of yoghurt

Fat	Temperature x Sources of milk			
	M₁ (Cow milk)		M₂ (Buffalo milk)	
	T₁ (39%)	T₂ (42%)	T₁ (39%)	T₂ (42%)
F₁ (4%)	1.02	1.01	1.02	1.01
F₂ (5%)	1.02	1.02	1.02	1.02
F₃ (6%)	1.01	1.02	1.02	1.02
Average	1.02	1.02	1.02	1.02

Not significant

Table 18.0 : The interaction effect of temperature, sources of milk and fat on lactic acid content (%) of yoghurt

Fat	Temperature x Sources of milk			
	M₁ (Cow milk)		M₂ (Buffalo milk)	
	T₁ (39%)	T₂ (42%)	T₁ (39%)	T₂ (42%)
F₁ (4%)	0.95	0.99	0.96	1.00
F₂ (5%)	0.96	0.99	0.96	1.00
F₃ (6%)	0.96	1.00	0.97	1.00
Average	0.96	0.99	0.96	1.00

Not significant

Table 18.1 : The interaction effect of temperature, sources of milk and fat on pH of yoghurt

Fat	Temperature x Sources of milk			
	M₁ (Cow milk)		M₂ (Buffalo milk)	
	T₁ (39%)	T₂ (42%)	T₁ (39%)	T₂ (42%)
F₁ (4%)	4.59	4.53	4.57	4.52
F₂ (5%)	4.58	4.53	4.57	4.52
F₃ (6%)	4.57	4.52	4.56	4.52
Average	4.58	4.53	4.57	4.52

Not significant

Table 18.2 : The interaction effect of temperature, sources of milk and SNF on fat content (%) of yoghurt

SNF	Temperature x Sources of milk			
	M_1 (Cow milk)		M_2 (Buffalo milk)	
	T_1 (39%)	T_2 (42%)	T_1 (39%)	T_2 (42%)
S_1 (10%)	5.02	5.01	5.01	5.02
S_2 (11%)	5.02	5.03	5.02	5.02
S_3 (12%)	5.01	5.02	5.02	5.02
Average	5.02	5.02	5.02	5.02

Not significant

Table 18.3 : The interaction effect of temperature, sources of milk and SNF on protein content (%) of yoghurt

SNF	Temperature x Sources of milk			
	M_1 (Cow milk)		M_2 (Buffalo milk)	
	T_1 (39%)	T_2 (42%)	T_1 (39%)	T_2 (42%)
S_1 (10%)	4.29	4.29	4.29	4.29
S_2 (11%)	4.67	4.67	4.67	4.67
S_3 (12%)	5.19	5.19	5.19	5.19
Average	4.72	4.72	4.72	4.72

Not significant

Table 18.4 : The interaction effect of temperature, sources of milk and SNF on lactose content (%) of yoghurt

SNF	Temperature x Sources of milk			
	M_1 (Cow milk)		M_2 (Buffalo milk)	
	T_1 (39%)	T_2 (42%)	T_1 (39%)	T_2 (42%)
S_1 (10%)	4.79	4.69	4.97	4.79
S_2 (11%)	5.22	5.15	5.39	5.25
S_3 (12%)	5.69	5.59	5.85	5.68
Average	5.23	5.14	5.40	5.24

Not significant

Table 18.5 : The interaction effect of temperature, sources of milk and SNF on ash content (%) of yoghurt

SNF	Temperature x Sources of milk			
	M_1 (Cow milk)		M_2 (Buffalo milk)	
	T_1 (39%)	T_2 (42%)	T_1 (39%)	T_2 (42%)
S_1 (10%)	0.88	0.88	0.88	0.88
S_2 (11%)	0.97	0.97	0.97	0.97
S_3 (12%)	1.20	1.20	1.21	1.02
Average	1.02	1.02	1.02	1.02

Not significant

Table 18.6 : The interaction effect of temperature, sources of milk and SNF on lactic acid content (%) of yoghurt

SNF	Temperature x Sources of milk			
	M_1 (Cow milk)		M_2 (Buffalo milk)	
	T_1 (39%)	T_2 (42%)	T_1 (39%)	T_2 (42%)
S_1 (10%)	0.91	0.96	0.92	0.96
S_2 (11%)	0.96	0.99	0.97	1.00
S_3 (12%)	0.99	1.03	1.00	1.04
Average	0.96	0.99	0.96	1.00

Not significant

Table 18.7 : The interaction effect of temperature, sources of milk and SNF on pH of yoghurt

SNF	Temperature x Sources of milk			
	M_1 (Cow milk)		M_2 (Buffalo milk)	
	T_1 (39%)	T_2 (42%)	T_1 (39%)	T_2 (42%)
S_1 (10%)	4.65	4.56	4.64	4.55
S_2 (11%)	4.56	4.53	4.54	4.52
S_3 (12%)	4.53	4.49	4.52	4.49
Average	4.58	4.53	4.57	4.52

Not significant

Table 18.8 : The interaction effect of temperature, sources of milk and starter culture on fat content (%) of yoghurt

| Starter Culture | Temperature x Sources of milk | | | |
| | M_1 (Cow milk) | | M_2 (Buffalo milk) | |
	T_1 (39%)	T_2 (42%)	T_1 (39%)	T_2 (42%)
Set₁ (SL 1:1)	5.04	5.03	5.02	5.02
Set₂ (SL 1:2)	5.00	5.01	5.01	5.01
Set₃ (SL 1:3)	5.02	5.02	5.02	5.02
Set₄ (SL 2:1)	5.02	5.03	5.04	5.03
Set₅ (SL 3:1)	5.01	5.01	5.01	5.02
Average	5.02	5.02	5.02	5.02

Not significant

Table 18.9 : The interaction effect of temperature, souces of milk and starter culture on protein content (%) of yoghurt

| Starter Culture | Temperature x Sources of milk | | | |
| | M_1 (Cow milk) | | M_2 (Buffalo milk) | |
	T_1 (39%)	T_2 (42%)	T_1 (39%)	T_2 (42%)
Set₁ (SL 1:1)	4.71	4.70	4.72	4.71
Set₂ (SL 1:2)	4.73	4.72	4.72	4.73
Set₃ (SL 1:3)	4.72	4.71	4.70	4.71
Set₄ (SL 2:1)	4.72	4.72	4.72	4.72
Set₅ (SL 3:1)	4.72	4.72	4.72	4.73
Average	4.72	4.72	4.72	4.72

Not significant

Table 19.0 : The interaction effect of temperature, sources of milk and starter culture on lactose (%) content of yoghurt

| Starter Culture | Temperature x Sources of milk | | | |
| | M_1 (Cow milk) | | M_2 (Buffalo milk) | |
	T_1 (39%)	T_2 (42%)	T_1 (39%)	T_2 (42%)
Set₁ (SL 1:1)	5.18	5.07	5.36	5.16
Set₂ (SL 1:2)	5.36	5.27	5.53	5.37
Set₃ (SL 1:3)	5.51	5.46	5.69	5.56
Set₄ (SL 2:1)	5.13	5.01	5.29	5.11
Set₅ (SL 3:1)	4.99	4.91	5.13	5.00
Average	5.23	5.14	5.40	5.24

Not significant

Table 19.1 : The interaction effect of temperature, sources of milk and starter culture on ash content (%) of yoghurt

Starter Culture	Temperature x Sources of milk			
	M_1 (Cow milk)		M_2 (Buffalo milk)	
	T_1 (39%)	T_2 (42%)	T_1 (39%)	T_2 (42%)
Set_1 (SL 1:1)	1.01	1.01	1.01	1.01
Set_2 (SL 1:2)	1.01	1.01	1.01	1.01
Set_3 (SL 1:3)	1.01	1.01	1.01	1.01
Set_4 (SL 2:1)	1.03	1.02	1.02	1.03
Set_5 (SL 3:1)	1.03	1.02	1.03	1.02
Average	1.02	1.02	1.02	1.02

Not significant

Table 19.2 : The interaction effect of temperature, sources of milk and starter culture on lactic acid content (%) of yoghurt

Starter Culture	Temperature x Sources of milk			
	M_1 (Cow milk)		M_2 (Buffalo milk)	
	T_1 (39%)	T_2 (42%)	T_1 (39%)	T_2 (42%)
Set_1 (SL 1:1)	0.87	0.90	0.88	0.90
Set_2 (SL 1:2)	0.88	0.91	0.89	0.91
Set_3 (SL 1:3)	0.89	0.93	0.91	0.94
Set_4 (SL 2:1)	1.06	1.09	1.06	1.10
Set_5 (SL 3:1)	1.07	1.14	1.08	1.14
Average	0.96	0.99	0.96	1.00

Not significant

Table 19.3 : The interaction effect of temperature, sources of milk and starter culture on pH of yoghurt

Starter Culture	Temperature x Sources of milk			
	M_1 (Cow milk)		M_2 (Buffalo milk)	
	T_1 (39%)	T_2 (42%)	T_1 (39%)	T_2 (42%)
Set_1 (SL 1:1)	4.68	4.60	4.66	4.59
Set_2 (SL 1:2)	4.64	4.58	4.62	4.58
Set_3 (SL 1:3)	4.62	4.56	4.60	4.56
Set_4 (SL 2:1)	4.48	4.47	4.49	4.46
Set_5 (SL 3:1)	4.47	4.41	4.46	4.41
Average	4.58	4.53	4.57	4.52

Not significant

Table 19.4 : The interaction effect of temperature, fat and SNF on fat content (%) of yoghurt

SNF	Temperature x Fat					
	T_1 (39°C)			T_2 (42°C)		
	F_1 (4%)	F_2 (5%)	F_3 (6%)	F_1 (4%)	F_2 (5%)	F_3 (6%)
S_1 (10%)	4.02	5.02	6.02	4.01	5.03	6.01
S_2 (11%)	4.04	5.00	6.04	4.04	5.01	6.04
S_3 (12%)	4.01	5.02	6.01	4.03	5.02	6.01
Average	4.02	5.01	6.02	4.03	5.02	6.02

Not significant

Table 19.5 : The interaction effect of temperature, fat and SNF on protein content (%) of yoghurt

SNF	Temperature x Fat					
	T_1 (39°C)			T_2 (42°C)		
	F_1 (4%)	F_2 (5%)	F_3 (6%)	F_1 (4%)	F_2 (5%)	F_3 (6%)
S_1 (10%)	4.29	4.29	4.29	4.29	4.29	4.29
S_2 (11%)	4.67	4.68	4.67	4.66	4.68	4.68
S_3 (12%)	5.19	5.19	5.19	5.19	5.19	5.19
Average	4.72	4.72	4.72	4.71	4.72	4.72

Not significant

Table 19.6 : The interaction effect of temperature, fat and SNF on lactose content (%) of yoghurt

SNF	Temperature x Fat					
	T_1 (39°C)			T_2 (42°C)		
	F_1 (4%)	F_2 (5%)	F_3 (6%)	F_1 (4%)	F_2 (5%)	F_3 (6%)
S_1 (10%)	4.90	4.92	4.81	4.77	4.78	4.67
S_2 (11%)	5.32	5.32	5.27	5.18	5.22	5.21
S_3 (12%)	5.79	5.77	5.75	5.59	5.69	5.62
Average	5.34	5.34	5.28	5.18	5.23	5.17

Not significant

Table 19.7 : The interaction effect of temperature, fat and SNF
on ash content (%) of yoghurt

| SNF | Temperature x Fat | | | | | |
| | T_1 (39°C) | | | T_2 (42°C) | | |
	F_1 (4%)	F_2 (5%)	F_3 (6%)	F_1 (4%)	F_2 (5%)	F_3 (6%)
S_1 (10%)	0.88	0.88	0.88	0.88	0.88	0.88
S_2 (11%)	0.97	0.97	0.97	0.97	0.98	0.97
S_3 (12%)	1.20	1.21	1.20	1.20	1.20	1.20
Average	1.02	1.02	1.02	1.01	1.02	1.02

Not significant

Table 19.8 : The interaction effect of temperature, fat and SNF
on lactic acid content(%) of yoghurt

| SNF | Temperature x Fat | | | | | |
| | T_1 (39°C) | | | T_2 (42°C) | | |
	F_1 (4%)	F_2 (5%)	F_3 (6%)	F_1 (4%)	F_2 (5%)	F_3 (6%)
S_1 (10%)	0.91	0.91	0.92	0.96	0.96	0.96
S_2 (11%)	0.96	0.97	0.97	1.00	1.00	1.00
S_3 (12%)	0.99	1.00	1.00	1.03	1.03	1.04
Average	0.96	0.96	0.96	0.99	1.00	1.00

Not significant

Table 19.9 : The interaction effect of temperature, fat and SNF
on pH of yoghurt

| SNF | Temperature x Fat | | | | | |
| | T_1 (39°C) | | | T_2 (42°C) | | |
	F_1 (4%)	F_2 (5%)	F_3 (6%)	F_1 (4%)	F_2 (5%)	F_3 (6%)
S_1 (10%)	4.66	4.64	4.63	4.56	4.56	4.55
S_2 (11%)	4.55	4.55	4.54	4.53	4.52	4.52
S_3 (12%)	4.53	4.52	4.52	4.50	4.49	4.49
Average	4.58	4.57	4.56	4.53	4.52	4.52

Not significant

Table 20.0 : The interaction effect of temperature, fat and
starter culture on fat content (%) of yoghurt

Starter Culture	Temperature x Fat					
	T_1 (39°C)			T_2 (42°C)		
	F_1 (4%)	F_2 (5%)	F_3 (6%)	F_1 (4%)	F_2 (5%)	F_3 (6%)
Set$_1$ (SL 1:1)	4.05	5.01	6.02	4.06	5.00	6.02
Set$_2$ (SL 1:2)	4.01	5.00	6.01	4.01	5.00	6.02
Set$_3$ (SL 1:3)	4.02	5.01	6.03	4.02	5.01	6.03
Set4 (SL 2:1)	4.03	5.03	6.03	4.04	5.03	6.02
Set5 (SL 3:1)	4.01	5.02	6.00	4.01	5.04	6.00
Average	4.02	5.01	6.02	4.03	5.02	6.02

Not significant

Table 20.1 : The interaction effect of temperature, fat and starter
culture on protein content (%) of yoghurt

Starter Culture	Temperature x Fat					
	T_1 (39°C)			T_2 (42°C)		
	F_1 (4%)	F_2 (5%)	F_3 (6%)	F_1 (4%)	F_2 (5%)	F_3 (6%)
Set$_1$ (SL 1:1)	4.70	4.72	4.71	4.69	4.71	4.72
Set$_2$ (SL 1:2)	4.73	4.73	4.72	4.73	4.72	4.73
Set$_3$ (SL 1:3)	4.71	4.71	4.71	4.71	4.72	4.71
Set4 (SL 2:1)	4.72	4.72	4.71	4.72	4.73	4.71
Set5 (SL 3:1)	4.72	4.72	4.72	4.73	4.72	4.72
Average	4.72	4.72	4.72	4.71	4.72	4.72

Not significant

Table 20.2 : The interaction effect of temperature, fat and starter
culture on lactose content (%) of yoghurt

Starter Culture	Temperature x Fat					
	T_1 (39°C)			T_2 (42°C)		
	F_1 (4%)	F_2 (5%)	F_3 (6%)	F_1 (4%)	F_2 (5%)	F_3 (6%)
Set$_1$ (SL 1:1)	5.30	5.27	5.23	5.08	5.15	5.12
Set$_2$ (SL 1:2)	5.47	5.45	5.43	5.32	5.37	5.28
Set$_3$ (SL 1:3)	5.62	5.62	5.56	5.55	5.54	5.45
Set4 (SL 2:1)	5.23	5.24	5.15	5.02	5.10	5.05
Set5 (SL 3:1)	5.07	5.10	5.02	4.93	5.00	4.93
Average	5.34	5.34	5.28	5.18	5.23	5.17

Not significant

Table 20.3 :   The interaction effect of temperature, fat and starter
culture on ash content (%) of yoghurt

Starter Culture	Temperature x Fat					
	T_1 (39^{0}C)			T_2 (42^{0}C)		
	F_1 (4%)	F_2 (5%)	F_3 (6%)	F_1 (4%)	F_2 (5%)	F_3 (6%)
Set$_1$ (SL 1:1)	1.02	1.02	1.00	1.00	1.01	1.02
Set$_2$ (SL 1:2)	1.01	1.02	1.02	1.01	1.01	1.01
Set$_3$ (SL 1:3)	1.01	1.02	1.01	1.01	1.01	1.01
Set4 (SL 2:1)	1.03	1.02	1.03	1.02	1.03	1.02
Set5 (SL 3:1)	1.03	1.03	1.02	1.02	1.02	1.02
Average	1.02	1.02	1.02	1.01	1.02	1.02

Not significant

Table 20.4 :   The interaction effect of temperature, fat and starter
culture on lactic acid content (%) of yoghurt

Starter Culture	Temperature x Fat					
	T_1 (39^{0}C)			T_2 (42^{0}C)		
	F_1 (4%)	F_2 (5%)	F_3 (6%)	F_1 (4%)	F_2 (5%)	F_3 (6%)
Set$_1$ (SL 1:1)	0.87	0.88	0.88	0.90	0.90	0.90
Set$_2$ (SL 1:2)	0.88	0.89	0.89	0.91	0.91	0.91
Set$_3$ (SL 1:3)	0.90	0.90	0.90	0.94	0.94	0.94
Set4 (SL 2:1)	1.05	1.06	1.06	1.09	1.09	1.10
Set5 (SL 3:1)	1.07	1.08	1.08	1.14	1.14	1.14
Average	0.96	0.96	0.96	0.99	1.00	1.00

Not significant

Table 20.5 :   The interaction effect of temperature, fat and
starter culture on pH of yoghurt

Starter Culture	Temperature x Fat					
	T_1 (39^{0}C)			T_2 (42^{0}C)		
	F_1 (4%)	F_2 (5%)	F_3 (6%)	F_1 (4%)	F_2 (5%)	F_3 (6%)
Set$_1$ (SL 1:1)	4.68	4.66	4.67	4.60	4.60	4.59
Set$_2$ (SL 1:2)	4.65	4.62	4.62	4.59	4.58	4.58
Set$_3$ (SL 1:3)	4.61	4.62	4.60	4.57	4.56	4.56
Set4 (SL 2:1)	4.50	4.49	4.47	4.47	4.46	4.46
Set5 (SL 3:1)	4.47	4.47	4.46	4.41	4.42	4.40
Average	4.58	4.57	4.56	4.53	4.52	4.52

Not significant

4.2.5.1 Interaction effects of temperature, SNF and starter culture on chemical attributes of yoghurt

Acidity

The lactic acid content of yoghurt enhanced significantly (P < 0.01) as the levels of SNF & temperature increases, except the values obtained between the interaction groups T_2 x S_1 x Set_1 and T_2 x S_2 x Set_1, T_2 x S_1 x Set_2 and T_2 x S_2 x Set_2, T_2 x S_2 x Set_4 and T_2 x S_3 Set_4, T_2 x S_2 x Set_5 and T_2 x S_3 x Set_5, irrespective of the culture were taken into account, it was noted that the acidity of yoghurt increased significantly (P < 0.01) as the proportion of lactobacilli increased to three fold in the milk containing 11% 12% of SNF incubated at 39°C & 42°C. When concentration of lactobacilli increased to two fold, the increase in acidity of yoghurt was statistically insignificant. Only in interaction groups T_1 x S_3 x Set_1 and T_1 x S_2 x Set_2 had significant (P < 0.01) effect on acidity of yoghurt. It was also observed that the acidity of yoghurt increased significantly (P < 0.01) as the concentration of streptococci increases in the milk having all the levels of SNF and temperature. The maximum acidity (1.15%) was recorded in interaction group T_2 x S_3 x Set_5 and the minimum value (0.85%) was observed in interaction group T_2 x S_1 x Set_1.

pH

The pH value of yoghurt reduced significantly (P <0.01) as the concentration of lactobacilli increases in the milk containing 10.0% SNF and incubated at 39°C (Table-21.1). Similarly, the pH value of yoghurt also reduced significantly (P < 0.01) when concentration of lactobacilli increased three fold in the milk containing 12% SNF sample incubated at 42°C.

The interaction effects of T x S x ST on fat (Table 20.6), protein (Table 20.7), lactose (Table 20.8) and ash (Table 20.9) content of yoghurt were statistically not significant.

Table 20.6 : The interaction effect of temperature, SNF and starter culture on fat content (%) of yoghurt

Starter Culture	Temperature x SNF					
	T_1 (39°C)			T_2 (42°C)		
	S_1 (10%)	S_2 (11%)	S_3 (12%)	S_1 (10%)	S_2 (11%)	S_3 (12%)
Set$_1$ (SL 1:1)	5.03	5.03	5.03	5.02	5.03	5.03
Set$_2$ (SL 1:2)	5.01	5.01	5.00	5.01	5.01	5.01
Set$_3$ (SL 1:3)	5.02	5.03	5.01	5.02	5.03	5.01
Set4 (SL 2:1)	5.02	5.04	5.03	5.02	5.04	5.04
Set5 (SL 3:1)	5.01	5.01	5.01	5.02	5.02	5.01
Average	5.02	5.02	5.01	5.02	5.03	5.02

Not significant

Table 20.7 : The interaction effect of temperature, SNF and starter culture on protein content (%) of yoghurt

Starter Culture	Temperature x SNF					
	T_1 (39°C)			T_2 (42°C)		
	S_1 (10%)	S_2 (11%)	S_3 (12%)	S_1 (10%)	S_2 (11%)	S_3 (12%)
Set$_1$ (SL 1:1)	4.03	4.66	5.18	4.30	4.64	5.18
Set$_2$ (SL 1:2)	4.28	4.70	5.20	4.29	4.69	5.20
Set$_3$ (SL 1:3)	4.30	4.64	5.19	4.30	4.64	5.19
Set4 (SL 2:1)	4.29	4.67	5.20	4.29	4.68	5.20
Set5 (SL 3:1)	4.29	4.68	5.18	4.29	4.70	5.18
Average	4.29	4.67	5.19	4.29	4.67	5.19

Not significant

Table 20.8 : The interaction effect of temperature, SNF and starter culture on lactose content (%) of yoghurt

Starter Culture	Temperature x SNF					
	T_1 (39°C)			T_2 (42°C)		
	S_1 (10%)	S_2 (11%)	S_3 (12%)	S_1 (10%)	S_2 (11%)	S_3 (12%)
Set$_1$ (SL 1:1)	4.87	5.18	5.75	4.71	5.08	5.55
Set$_2$ (SL 1:2)	4.99	5.37	5.98	4.83	5.28	5.85
Set$_3$ (SL 1:3)	5.13	5.58	6.08	5.02	5.51	5.02
Set4 (SL 2:1)	4.77	5.29	5.57	4.62	5.12	5.43
Set5 (SL 3:1)	4.63	5.08	5.47	4.52	5.03	5.32
Average	4.88	5.30	5.77	4.74	5.20	5.63

Not significant

Table 20.9 : The interaction effect of temperature, SNF and starter culture on ash content (%) of yoghurt

Starter Culture	Temperature x SNF					
	T_1 (39°C)			T_2 (42°C)		
	S_1 (10%)	S_2 (11%)	S_3 (12%)	S_1 (10%)	S_2 (11%)	S_3 (12%)
Set₁ (SL 1:1)	0.87	0.97	1.20	0.88	0.97	1.19
Set₂ (SL 1:2)	0.88	0.97	1.20	0.88	0.97	1.19
Set₃ (SL 1:3)	0.87	0.97	1.20	0.87	0.97	1.19
Set4 (SL 2:1)	0.88	0.97	1.22	0.88	0.97	1.22
Set5 (SL 3:1)	0.89	0.98	1.21	0.88	0.98	1.21
Average	0.88	0.97	1.20	0.88	0.97	1.20

Not significant

Table 21.0 : The interaction effect of temperature, SNF and starter culture on lactic acid content (%) of yoghurt

Starter Culture	Temperature x SNF					
	T_1 (39°C)			T_2 (42°C)		
	S_1 (10%)	S_2 (11%)	S_3 (12%)	S_1 (10%)	S_2 (11%)	S_3 (12%)
Set₁ (SL 1:1)	0.85	0.87	0.90	0.87	0.88	0.95
Set₂ (SL 1:2)	0.86	0.88	0.92	0.88	0.89	0.96
Set₃ (SL 1:3)	0.86	0.91	0.93	0.88	0.95	0.98
Set4 (SL 2:1)	0.99	1.08	1.10	1.03	1.12	1.13
Set5 (SL 3:1)	1.01	1.10	1.13	1.13	1.14	1.15
Average	0.91	0.97	1.00	0.96	1.00	1.03

CD at 5% = 0.014 at 1% = 0.019

Table 21.1 : The interaction effect of temperature, SNF and starter culture on pH of yoghurt

Starter Culture	Temperature x SNF					
	T_1 (39°C)			T_2 (42°C)		
	S_1 (10%)	S_2 (11%)	S_3 (12%)	S_1 (10%)	S_2 (11%)	S_3 (12%)
Set₁ (SL 1:1)	4.79	4.63	4.59	4.63	4.61	4.56
Set₂ (SL 1:2)	4.71	4.61	4.58	4.61	4.59	4.55
Set₃ (SL 1:3)	4.66	4.61	4.57	4.60	4.55	4.54
Set4 (SL 2:1)	4.54	4.45	4.47	4.51	4.45	4.43
Set5 (SL 3:1)	4.53	4.44	4.43	4.43	4.41	4.39
Average	4.65	4.55	4.53	4.55	4.52	4.49

CD at 5% = 0.026 at 1% = 0.035

The combined effects of F x M x S, F x M x ST, F x S x ST, S x M x ST, T x M x F x S, T x M x F x ST, T x M x S x ST, T x F x S x ST, F x M x S x ST, T x M x F x S x ST on fat, protein, lactose, ash and acidity and pH values of yoghurt samples were statistically not significant (Table-21.2 – 27.1).

Table 21.2 : The interaction effect of fat, source of milk and SNF on fat content (%) of yoghurt

SNF	Sources of milk x Fat					
	M_1 (Cow milk)			M_2 (Buffalo milk)		
	F_1 (4%)	F_2 (5%)	F_3 (6%)	F_1 (4%)	F_2 (5%)	F_3 (6%)
S_1 (10%)	4.02	5.03	6.01	4.02	5.02	6.02
S_2 (11%)	4.05	5.00	6.04	4.03	5.01	6.04
S_3 (12%)	4.02	5.02	6.01	4.02	5.02	6.01
Average	4.03	5.02	6.02	4.02	5.02	6.02

Not significant

Table 21.3 : The interaction effect of fat, source of milk and SNF on protein content (%) of yoghurt

SNF	Sources of milk x Fat					
	M_1 (Cow milk)			M_2 (Buffalo milk)		
	F_1 (4%)	F_2 (5%)	F_3 (6%)	F_1 (4%)	F_2 (5%)	F_3 (6%)
S_1 (10%)	4.29	4.29	4.29	4.29	4.29	4.29
S_2 (11%)	4.66	4.68	4.68	4.67	4.68	4.67
S_3 (12%)	5.19	5.19	5.19	5.19	5.19	5.19
Average	4.71	4.72	4.72	4.72	4.72	4.72

Not significant

Table 21.4 : The interaction effect of fat, source of milk and SNF on lactose content (%) of yoghurt

SNF	Sources of milk x Fat					
	M_1 (Cow milk)			M_2 (Buffalo milk)		
	F_1 (4%)	F_2 (5%)	F_3 (6%)	F_1 (4%)	F_2 (5%)	F_3 (6%)
S_1 (10%)	4.76	4.78	4.68	4.91	4.93	4.80
S_2 (11%)	5.18	5.20	5.19	5.33	5.35	5.29
S_3 (12%)	5.62	5.66	5.94	5.76	5.81	5.73
Average	5.19	5.21	5.17	5.33	5.36	5.27

Not significant

Table 21.5 : The interaction effect of fat, source of milk and SNF on ash content (%) of yoghurt

SNF	Sources of milk x Fat					
	M_1 (Cow milk)			M_2 (Buffalo milk)		
	F_1 (4%)	F_2 (5%)	F_3 (6%)	F_1 (4%)	F_2 (5%)	F_3 (6%)
S_1 (10%)	0.88	0.88	0.88	0.88	0.88	0.88
S_2 (11%)	0.98	0.97	0.97	0.97	0.97	0.97
S_3 (12%)	1.20	1.21	1.20	1.20	1.21	1.20
Average	1.02	1.02	1.02	1.02	1.02	1.02

Not significant

Table 21.6 : The interaction effect of fat, source of milk and SNF on lactic acid content of yoghurt

SNF	Sources of milk x Fat					
	M_1 (Cow milk)			M_2 (Buffalo milk)		
	F_1 (4%)	F_2 (5%)	F_3 (6%)	F_1 (4%)	F_2 (5%)	F_3 (6%)
S_1 (10%)	0.94	0.93	0.94	0.93	0.94	0.94
S_2 (11%)	0.98	0.98	0.98	0.99	0.99	0.99
S_3 (12%)	1.01	1.01	1.01	1.01	1.02	1.02
Average	0.97	0.97	0.98	0.98	0.98	0.98

Not significant

Table 21.7 : The interaction effect o fat, source of milk and SNF on pH of yoghurt

SNF	Sources of milk x Fat					
	M_1 (Cow milk)			M_2 (Buffalo milk)		
	F_1 (4%)	F_2 (5%)	F_3 (6%)	F_1 (4%)	F_2 (5%)	F_3 (6%)
S_1 (10%)	4.62	4.60	4.60	4.60	4.60	4.59
S_2 (11%)	4.54	4.55	4.54	4.53	4.53	4.52
S_3 (12%)	4.52	4.51	4.51	4.52	4.51	4.50
Average	4.56	4.55	4.55	4.55	4.54	4.54

Not significant

Table 21.8 :   The interaction effect of fat, sources of milk and
starter culture on fat content (%) of yoghurt

| Starter Culture | Fat x Sources of milk | | | | | |
| | M_1 (Cow milk) | | | M_2 (Buffallo milk) | | |
	F_1 (4%)	F_2 (5%)	F_3 (6%)	F_1 (4%)	F_2 (5%)	F_3 (6%)
Set$_1$ (SL 1:1)	4.08	5.00	6.02	4.03	5.01	6.03
Set$_2$ (SL 1:2)	4.01	5.00	6.01	4.01	5.00	6.02
Set$_3$ (SL 1:3)	4.02	5.01	6.03	4.02	5.01	6.03
Set4 (SL 2:1)	4.03	5.03	6.02	4.04	5.03	6.03
Set5 (SL 3:1)	4.01	5.03	6.00	4.01	5.03	6.00
Average	4.03	5.02	6.02	4.02	5.02	6.02

Not significant

Table 21.9 :   The interaction effect of fat, sources of milk and starter
culture on protein content (%) of yoghurt

| Starter Culture | Fat x Sources of milk | | | | | |
| | M_1 (Cow milk) | | | M_2 (Buffallo milk) | | |
	F_1 (4%)	F_2 (5%)	F_3 (6%)	F_1 (4%)	F_2 (5%)	F_3 (6%)
Set$_1$ (SL 1:1)	4.69	4.71	4.71	4.70	4.73	4.72
Set$_2$ (SL 1:2)	4.73	4.72	4.73	4.73	4.73	4.73
Set$_3$ (SL 1:3)	4.71	4.72	4.72	4.70	4.71	4.71
Set4 (SL 2:1)	4.71	4.73	4.72	4.73	4.72	4.71
Set5 (SL 3:1)	4.72	4.72	4.72	4.73	4.72	4.72
Average	4.71	4.72	4.72	4.72	4.72	4.72

Not significant

Table 22.0 :   The interaction effect of fat, sources of milk and starter
culture on lactose content (%) of yoghurt

| Starter Culture | Fat x Sources of milk | | | | | |
| | M_1 (Cow milk) | | | M_2 (Buffallo milk) | | |
	F_1 (4%)	F_2 (5%)	F_3 (6%)	F_1 (4%)	F_2 (5%)	F_3 (6%)
Set$_1$ (SL 1:1)	5.12	5.14	5.12	5.26	5.29	5.23
Set$_2$ (SL 1:2)	5.32	5.33	5.03	5.47	5.48	5.41
Set$_3$ (SL 1:3)	5.50	5.50	5.45	5.67	5.65	5.56
Set4 (SL 2:1)	5.05	5.10	5.05	5.20	5.25	5.15
Set5 (SL 3:1)	4.94	4.98	4.93	5.06	5.13	5.02
Average	5.19	5.21	5.17	5.33	5.36	5.27

Not significant

Table 22.1 : The interaction effect of fat, sources of milk and starter culture on ash content (%) of yoghurt

Starter Culture	Fat x Sources of milk					
	M_1 (Cow milk)			M_2 (Buffallo milk)		
	F_1 (4%)	F_2 (5%)	F_3 (6%)	F_1 (4%)	F_2 (5%)	F_3 (6%)
Set$_1$ (SL 1:1)	1.01	1.01	1.01	1.01	1.02	1.01
Set$_2$ (SL 1:2)	1.01	1.02	1.01	1.01	1.01	1.02
Set$_3$ (SL 1:3)	1.01	1.02	1.01	1.01	1.01	1.01
Set4 (SL 2:1)	1.02	1.03	1.02	1.03	1.02	1.03
Set5 (SL 3:1)	1.03	1.03	1.02	1.02	1.03	1.03
Average	1.02	1.02	1.02	1.02	1.02	1.02

Not significant

Table 22.2 : The interaction effect of fat, sources of milk and starter culture on lactic acid content (%) of yoghurt

Starter Culture	Fat x Sources of milk					
	M_1 (Cow milk)			M_2 (Buffallo milk)		
	F_1 (4%)	F_2 (5%)	F_3 (6%)	F_1 (4%)	F_2 (5%)	F_3 (6%)
Set$_1$ (SL 1:1)	0.88	0.89	0.89	0.89	0.89	0.89
Set$_2$ (SL 1:2)	0.89	0.90	0.90	0.90	0.90	0.90
Set$_3$ (SL 1:3)	0.91	0.91	0.92	0.92	0.92	0.93
Set4 (SL 2:1)	1.07	1.07	1.08	1.08	1.08	1.98
Set5 (SL 3:1)	1.10	1.10	1.11	1.11	1.11	1.12
Average	0.97	0.97	0.98	0.98	0.98	0.98

Not significant

Table 22.3 : The interaction effect of fat, sources of milk and starter culture on pH of yoghurt

Starter Culture	Fat x Sources of milk					
	M_1 (Cow milk)			M_2 (Buffallo milk)		
	F_1 (4%)	F_2 (5%)	F_3 (6%)	F_1 (4%)	F_2 (5%)	F_3 (6%)
Set$_1$ (SL 1:1)	4.65	4.63	4.64	4.63	4.63	4.62
Set$_2$ (SL 1:2)	4.63	4.61	4.60	4.60	4.60	4.60
Set$_3$ (SL 1:3)	4.59	4.61	4.59	4.59	4.58	4.58
Set4 (SL 2:1)	4.49	4.47	4.47	4.48	4.48	4.46
Set5 (SL 3:1)	4.44	4.44	4.44	4.44	4.44	4.43
Average	4.56	4.55	4.55	4.55	4.54	4.54

Not significant

Table 22.4 : The interaction effect of fat, SNF and starter culture on fat content (%) of yoghurt

Starter culture	Fat x SNF								
	F_1 (4%)			F_2 (5%)			F_3 (6%)		
	S_1 (10%)	S_2 (11%)	S_3 (12%)	S_1 (10%)	S_2 (11%)	S_3 (12%)	S_1 (10%)	S_2 (11%)	S_3 (12%)
Set$_1$ (SL 1:1)	4.04	4.06	4.08	5.01	5.00	5.01	6.03	6.03	6.01
Set$_2$ (SL 1:2)	4.00	4.02	4.00	5.00	5.00	5.01	6.03	6.01	6.01
Set$_3$ (SL 1:3)	4.05	4.00	4.00	5.00	5.00	5.03	6.00	6.10	6.00
Set$_4$ (SL 2:1)	4.00	4.08	4.03	5.05	5.01	5.04	6.01	6.04	6.03
Set$_5$ (SL 3:1)	4.00	4.03	4.00	5.05	5.01	5.02	6.00	6.00	6.00
Average	4.02	4.04	4.02	5.02	5.00	5.02	6.01	6.04	6.01

Not significant

Table 22.5 : The interaction effect of fat, SNF and starter culture on protein content (%) of yoghurt

Starter culture	Fat x SNF								
	F_1 (4%)			F_2 (5%)			F_3 (6%)		
	S_1 (10%)	S_2 (11%)	S_3 (12%)	S_1 (10%)	S_2 (11%)	S_3 (12%)	S_1 (10%)	S_2 (11%)	S_3 (12%)
Set$_1$ (SL 1:1)	4.30	4.61	5.18	4.30	4.68	5.18	4.30	4.66	5.18
Set$_2$ (SL 1:2)	4.28	4.70	5.20	4.28	4.69	5.20	4.29	4.70	5.20
Set$_3$ (SL 1:3)	4.30	4.63	5.20	4.30	4.65	5.19	4.30	4.65	5.19
Set$_4$ (SL 2:1)	4.29	4.68	5.20	4.29	4.69	5.20	4.29	4.65	5.20
Set$_5$ (SL 3:1)	4.29	4.70	5.18	4.29	4.69	5.19	4.30	4.69	5.18
Average	4.29	4.66	5.19	4.29	4.68	5.19	4.29	4.67	5.19

Not significant

Table 22.6 : The interaction effect of fat, SNF and starter culture on lactose content (%) of yoghurt

Starter culture	Fat x SNF								
	F_1 (4%)			F_2 (5%)			F_3 (6%)		
	S_1 (10%)	S_2 (11%)	S_3 (12%)	S_1 (10%)	S_2 (11%)	S_3 (12%)	S_1 (10%)	S_2 (11%)	S_3 (12%)
Set$_1$ (SL 1:1)	4.81	5.13	5.63	4.84	5.13	5.68	4.73	5.15	5.65
Set$_2$ (SL 1:2)	4.93	5.33	5.93	4.95	5.35	5.93	4.86	5.03	5.90
Set$_3$ (SL 1:3)	5.10	5.58	6.08	5.10	5.56	5.08	5.01	5.50	6.00
Set$_4$ (SL 2:1)	4.73	5.18	5.48	4.75	5.24	5.53	4.60	5.20	5.50
Set$_5$ (SL 3:1)	4.60	5.05	5.35	4.63	5.08	5.45	4.50	5.05	5.38
Average	4.83	5.25	5.69	4.85	5.27	5.73	4.74	5.24	5.69

Not significant

Table 22.7 : The interaction effect of fat, SNF and starter culture on ash content (%) of yoghurt

Starter culture	Fat x SNF								
	F_1 (4%)			F_2 (5%)			F_3 (6%)		
	S_1 (10%)	S_2 (11%)	S_3 (12%)	S_1 (10%)	S_2 (11%)	S_3 (12%)	S_1 (10%)	S_2 (11%)	S_3 (12%)
Set_1 (SL 1:1)	0.87	0.97	1.19	0.88	0.97	1.02	0.87	0.97	1.19
Set_2 (SL 1:2)	0.88	0.97	1.19	0.88	0.97	1.19	0.88	0.97	1.20
Set_3 (SL 1:3)	0.87	0.98	1.19	0.87	0.97	1.20	0.87	0.97	1.19
Set_4 (SL 2:1)	0.89	0.97	1.22	0.88	0.97	1.23	0.88	0.97	1.23
Set_5 (SL 3:1)	0.89	0.98	1.21	0.89	0.96	1.21	0.88	0.98	1.21
Average	0.88	0.97	1.20	0.88	0.96	1.21	0.88	0.97	1.20

Not significant

Table 22.8 : The interaction effect of fat, SNF and starter culture on lactic acid content (%) of yoghurt

Starter culture	Fat x SNF								
	F_1 (4%)			F_2 (5%)			F_3 (6%)		
	S_1 (10%)	S_2 (11%)	S_3 (12%)	S_1 (10%)	S_2 (11%)	S_3 (12%)	S_1 (10%)	S_2 (11%)	S_3 (12%)
Set_1 (SL 1:1)	0.86	0.88	0.92	0.86	0.88	0.93	0.86	0.88	0.93
Set_2 (SL 1:2)	0.87	0.89	0.93	0.87	0.89	0.94	0.87	0.89	0.94
Set_3 (SL 1:3)	0.87	0.93	0.95	0.87	0.93	0.95	0.88	0.93	0.96
Set_4 (SL 2:1)	1.01	1.10	1.11	1.01	1.11	1.12	1.01	1.11	1.12
Set_5 (SL 3:1)	1.07	1.12	1.13	1.06	1.12	1.14	1.07	1.12	1.15
Average	0.94	0.98	1.01	0.94	0.98	1.01	0.94	0.99	1.02

Not significant

Table 22.9 : The interaction effect of fat, SNF and starter culture on pH of yoghurt

Starter culture	Fat x SNF								
	F_1 (4%)			F_2 (5%)			F_3 (6%)		
	S_1 (10%)	S_2 (11%)	S_3 (12%)	S_1 (10%)	S_2 (11%)	S_3 (12%)	S_1 (10%)	S_2 (11%)	S_3 (12%)
Set_1 (SL 1:1)	4.73	4.62	4.58	4.70	4.62	4.57	4.69	4.63	4.57
Set_2 (SL 1:2)	4.69	4.60	4.57	4.65	4.60	4.56	4.64	4.60	4.56
Set_3 (SL 1:3)	4.63	4.58	4.56	4.63	4.60	4.55	4.63	4.57	4.55
Set_4 (SL 2:1)	4.53	4.47	4.47	4.53	4.45	4.45	4.53	4.44	4.43
Set_5 (SL 3:1)	4.46	4.43	4.42	4.49	4.43	4.41	4.48	4.42	4.40
Average	4.61	4.54	4.52	4.69	4.54	4.51	4.59	4.53	4.50

Not significant

Table 23.0 :   The interaction effect of SNF, sources of milk and starter culture on fat content (%) of yoghurt

Starter culture	SNF x Sources of milk					
	M_1 (Cow milk)			M_2 (Buffalo milk)		
	S_1 (10%)	S_2 (11%)	S_3 (12%)	S_1 (10%)	S_2 (11%)	S_3 (12%)
Set_1 (SL 1:1)	5.03	5.04	5.03	5.02	5.01	5.03
Set_2 (SL 1:2)	5.01	5.01	5.00	5.01	5.01	5.01
Set_3 (SL 1:3)	5.02	5.03	5.01	5.02	5.03	5.01
Set_4 (SL 2:1)	5.02	5.04	5.03	5.02	5.04	5.04
Set_5 (SL 3:1)	5.02	5.01	5.01	5.01	5.02	5.01
Average	5.02	5.03	5.02	5.02	5.02	5.02

Not significant

Table 23.1 : The interaction effect of SNF, sources of milk and starter culture on protein content (%) of yoghurt

Starter culture	SNF x Sources of milk					
	M_1 (Cow milk)			M_2 (Buffalo milk)		
	S_1 (10%)	S_2 (11%)	S_3 (12%)	S_1 (10%)	S_2 (11%)	S_3 (12%)
Set_1 (SL 1:1)	4.30	4.63	5.18	4.30	4.67	5.18
Set_2 (SL 1:2)	4.29	4.69	5.20	4.28	4.70	5.20
Set_3 (SL 1:3)	4.30	4.66	5.19	4.30	4.63	5.19
Set_4 (SL 2:1)	4.28	4.68	5.20	4.29	4.67	5.20
Set_5 (SL 3:1)	4.29	4.69	5.18	4.29	4.69	5.18
Average	4.29	4.67	5.19	4.29	4.67	5.19

Not significant

Table 23.2 :   The interaction effect of SNF, sources of milk and starter culture on lactose content (%) of yoghurt

Starter culture	SNF x Sources of milk					
	M_1 (Cow milk)			M_2 (Buffalo milk)		
	S_1 (10%)	S_2 (11%)	S_3 (12%)	S_1 (10%)	S_2 (11%)	S_3 (12%)
Set_1 (SL 1:1)	4.72	5.07	5.58	4.86	5.20	5.72
Set_2 (SL 1:2)	4.84	5.26	5.85	4.98	5.39	5.98
Set_3 (SL 1:3)	4.99	5.48	5.98	5.15	5.61	6.12
Set_4 (SL 2:1)	4.63	5.14	5.43	4.76	5.27	5.57
Set_5 (SL 3:1)	4.52	4.99	5.34	4.63	5.13	5.44
Average	4.74	5.19	5.64	4.88	5.32	5.77

Not significant

Table 23.3 :   The interaction effect of SNF, sources of milk and
                starter culture on ash content (%) of yoghurt

Starter culture	SNF x Sources of milk					
	M₁ (Cow milk)			M₂ (Buffalo milk)		
	S₁ (10%)	S₂ (11%)	S₃ (12%)	S₁ (10%)	S₂ (11%)	S₃ (12%)
Set₁ (SL 1:1)	0.87	0.97	1.19	0.88	0.97	1.19
Set₂ (SL 1:2)	0.88	0.97	1.19	0.88	0.97	1.20
Set₃ (SL 1:3)	0.87	0.97	1.20	0.87	0.97	1.19
Set₄ (SL 2:1)	0.88	0.97	1.22	0.88	0.97	1.22
Set₅ (SL 3:1)	0.89	0.98	1.21	0.89	0.98	1.21
Average	0.89	0.97	1.20	0.88	0.97	1.20

Not significant

Table 23.4 :   The interaction effect of SNF, sources of milk and starter
                culture on lactic acid content (%) of yoghurt

Starter culture	SNF x Sources of milk					
	M₁ (Cow milk)			M₂ (Buffalo milk)		
	S₁ (10%)	S₂ (11%)	S₃ (12%)	S₁ (10%)	S₂ (11%)	S₃ (12%)
Set₁ (SL 1:1)	0.86	0.88	0.92	0.87	0.88	0.93
Set₂ (SL 1:2)	0.87	0.88	0.93	0.87	0.89	0.94
Set₃ (SL 1:3)	0.87	0.93	0.95	0.88	0.94	0.96
Set₄ (SL 2:1)	1.01	1.01	1.12	1.02	1.11	1.12
Set₅ (SL 3:1)	1.07	1.11	1.13	1.06	1.13	1.15
Average	0.94	0.98	1.01	0.94	0.99	1.02

Not significant

Table 23.5 :   The interaction effect of SNF, sources of milk and
                starter culture on pH of yoghurt

Starter culture	SNF x Sources of milk					
	M₁ (Cow milk)			M₂ (Buffalo milk)		
	S₁ (10%)	S₂ (11%)	S₃ (12%)	S₁ (10%)	S₂ (11%)	S₃ (12%)
Set₁ (SL 1:1)	4.72	4.63	4.58	4.70	4.61	4.57
Set₂ (SL 1:2)	4.67	4.60	4.57	4.65	4.59	4.56
Set₃ (SL 1:3)	4.64	4.59	4.56	4.63	4.57	4.55
Set₄ (SL 2:1)	4.53	4.46	4.44	4.52	4.44	4.46
Set₅ (SL 3:1)	4.47	4.43	4.41	4.48	4.42	4.40
Average	4.60	4.54	4.51	4.60	4.53	4.51

Not significant

Table 23.6 : The interaction effect of sources of milk, temperature, fat and SNF on fat content (%) of yoghurt

SNF	Sources of milk x Temperature x Fat											
	M_1 (Cow milk)						M_2 (Buffalo milk)					
	T_1 (39°C)			T_2 (42°C)			T_1 (39°C)			T_2 (42°C)		
	F_1 (4%)	F_2 (5%)	F_3 (6%)	F_1 (4%)	F_2 (5%)	F_3 (6%)	F_1 (4%)	F_2 (5%)	F_3 (6%)	F_1 (4%)	F_2 (5%)	F_3 (6%)
S1 (10%)	4.03	5.02	6.02	4.01	5.03	6.01	4.01	5.01	6.01	4.02	5.02	6.02
S2 (11%)	4.04	5.00	6.03	4.05	5.00	6.04	4.03	5.00	6.04	4.03	5.01	6.03
S3 (12%)	4.02	5.01	6.00	4.02	5.02	6.01	4.00	5.03	6.02	4.03	5.02	6.01
Average	4.03	5.01	6.02	4.03	5.02	6.02	4.02	5.02	6.02	4.02	5.02	6.02

Not significant

Table 23.7 : The interaction effect of sources of milk, temperature, fat and SNF on protein content (%) of yoghurt

SNF	Sources of milk x Temperature x Fat											
	M_1 (Cow milk)						M_2 (Buffalo milk)					
	T_1 (39°C)			T_2 (42°C)			T_1 (39°C)			T_2 (42°C)		
	F_1 (4%)	F_2 (5%)	F_3 (6%)	F_1 (4%)	F_2 (5%)	F_3 (6%)	F_1 (4%)	F_2 (5%)	F_3 (6%)	F_1 (4%)	F_2 (5%)	F_3 (6%)
S1 (10%)	4.29	4.29	4.29	4.29	4.29	4.29	4.29	4.29	4.29	4.29	4.29	4.29
S2 (11%)	4.66	4.63	4.61	4.66	4.66	4.68	4.67	4.67	4.66	4.66	4.63	4.67
S3 (12%)	5.19	5.19	5.19	5.19	5.19	5.19	5.19	5.19	5.19	5.19	5.19	5.19
Average	4.71	4.72	4.72	4.71	4.71	4.72	4.72	4.72	4.71	4.72	4.72	4.72

Not significant

Table 23.8 : The interaction effect of sources of milk, temperature, fat and SNF on lactose content (%) of yoghurt

SNF	Sources of milk x Temperature x Fat											
	M₁ (Cow milk)						M₂ (Buffalo milk)					
	T₁ (39⁰C)			T₂ (42⁰C)			T₁ (39⁰C)			T₂ (42⁰C)		
	F_1 (4%)	F_2 (5%)	F_3 (6%)	F_1 (4%)	F_2 (5%)	F_3 (6%)	F_1 (4%)	F_2 (5%)	F_3 (6%)	F_1 (4%)	F_2 (5%)	F_3 (6%)
S1 (10%)	4.80	4.82	4.74	4.72	4.73	4.62	5.00	5.02	4.88	4.81	4.83	4.72
S2 (11%)	5.22	5.22	5.22	5.13	5.17	5.16	5.42	5.42	5.32	5.23	5.27	5.26
S3 (12%)	5.70	5.67	5.70	5.54	5.64	5.58	5.88	5.87	5.80	5.64	5.74	5.66
Average	5.24	5.24	5.22	5.13	5.18	5.12	5.43	5.44	5.33	5.23	5.82	5.87

Not significant

Table 23.9 : The interaction effect of sources of milk, temperature, fat and SNF on ash content (%) of yoghurt

SNF	Sources of milk x Temperature x Fat											
	M₁ (Cow milk)						M₂ (Buffalo milk)					
	T₁ (39⁰C)			T₂ (42⁰C)			T₁ (39⁰C)			T₂ (42⁰C)		
	F_1 (4%)	F_2 (5%)	F_3 (6%)	F_1 (4%)	F_2 (5%)	F_3 (6%)	F_1 (4%)	F_2 (5%)	F_3 (6%)	F_1 (4%)	F_2 (5%)	F_3 (6%)
S1 (10%)	0.88	0.88	0.88	0.87	0.88	0.87	0.88	0.87	0.87	0.88	0.88	0.88
S2 (11%)	0.98	0.97	0.97	0.97	0.97	0.97	0.96	0.97	0.97	0.97	0.98	0.97
S3 (12%)	1.20	1.21	1.19	1.20	1.20	1.21	1.20	1.21	1.20	1.19	1.20	1.20
Average	1.02	1.02	1.01	1.01	1.02	1.02	1.02	1.02	1.02	1.01	1.02	1.02

Not significant

Table 24.0 : The interaction effect of sources of milk, temperature, fat and SNF on lactic acid content (%) of yoghurt

SNF	Sources of milk x Temperature x Fat											
	M₁ (Cow milk)						M₂ (Buffalo milk)					
	T_1 (39°C)			T_2 (42°C)			T_1 (39°C)			T_2 (42°C)		
	F_1 (4%)	F_2 (5%)	F_3 (6%)	F_1 (4%)	F_2 (5%)	F_3 (6%)	F_1 (4%)	F_2 (5%)	F_3 (6%)	F_1 (4%)	F_2 (5%)	F_3 (6%)
S1 (10%)	0.91	0.91	0.91	0.96	0.96	0.96	0.91	0.92	0.92	0.96	0.96	0.96
S2 (11%)	0.96	0.97	0.97	0.99	0.99	1.00	0.97	0.97	0.97	1.00	1.00	1.01
S3 (12%)	0.99	0.99	0.99	1.02	1.03	1.03	1.00	1.00	1.00	1.03	1.04	1.04
Average	0.95	0.96	0.96	0.99	0.99	1.00	0.96	0.96	0.97	1.00	1.00	1.00

Not significant

Table 24.1 : The interaction effect of sources of milk, temperature fat and SNF on pH of yoghurt

SNF	Sources of milk x Temperature x Fat											
	M₁ (Cow milk)						M₂ (Buffalo milk)					
	T_1 (39°C)			T_2 (42°C)			T_1 (39°C)			T_2 (42°C)		
	F_1 (4%)	F_2 (5%)	F_3 (6%)	F_1 (4%)	F_2 (5%)	F_3 (6%)	F_1 (4%)	F_2 (5%)	F_3 (6%)	F_1 (4%)	F_2 (5%)	F_3 (6%)
S1 (10%)	4.68	4.65	4.64	4.56	4.56	4.56	4.64	4.64	4.63	4.55	4.55	4.55
S2 (11%)	4.55	4.57	4.56	4.54	4.52	4.52	4.54	4.54	4.53	4.52	4.52	4.51
S3 (12%)	4.54	4.52	4.52	4.50	4.49	4.49	4.53	4.53	4.51	4.50	4.49	4.49
Average	4.59	4.58	4.57	4.53	4.53	4.52	4.57	4.57	4.56	4.52	4.52	4.52

Not significant

Table 24.2 : The interaction effect of sources of milk, temperature, fat and starter culture on fat content (%) of yoghurt

Starter Culture	Sources of milk x Temperature x Fat											
	M₁ (Cow milk)						M₂ (Buffalo milk)					
	T₁ (39°C)			T₂ (42°C)			T₁ (39°C)			T₂ (42°C)		
	F₁ (4%)	F₂ (5%)	F₃ (6%)	F₁ (4%)	F₂ (5%)	F₃ (6%)	F₁ (4%)	F₂ (5%)	F₃ (6%)	F₁ (4%)	F₂ (5%)	F₃ (6%)
Set1 (SL 1:1)	4.10	5.00	6.02	4.07	5.01	6.02	4.01	5.02	6.03	4.05	5.00	6.02
Set2 (SL 1:2)	4.00	5.00	6.01	4.01	5.00	6.01	4.01	5.00	6.01	4.00	5.01	6.03
Set3 (SL 1:3)	4.02	5.00	6.03	4.02	5.02	6.03	4.02	5.02	6.03	4.02	5.00	6.03
Set4(SL 2:1)	4.03	5.03	6.01	4.03	5.03	6.03	4.03	5.03	6.04	4.05	5.03	6.01
Set5 (SL 3:1)	4.01	5.03	6.00	4.01	5.03	6.00	4.01	5.01	6.00	4.01	5.04	6.00
Average	4.03	5.01	6.02	4.03	5.02	6.02	4.02	5.02	6.02	4.02	5.02	6.02

Not significant

Table 24.3 : The interaction effect of sources of milk, temperature, fat and starter culture on protein content (%) of yoghurt

Starter Culture	Sources of milk x Temperature x Fat											
	M₁ (Cow milk)						M₂ (Buffalo milk)					
	T₁ (39°C)			T₂ (42°C)			T₁ (39°C)			T₂ (42°C)		
	F₁ (4%)	F₂ (5%)	F₃ (6%)	F₁ (4%)	F₂ (5%)	F₃ (6%)	F₁ (4%)	F₂ (5%)	F₃ (6%)	F₁ (4%)	F₂ (5%)	F₃ (6%)
Set1 (SL 1:1)	4.69	4.72	4.71	4.69	4.69	4.71	4.71	4.73	4.71	4.69	4.72	4.73
Set2 (SL 1:2)	4.73	4.73	4.72	4.73	4.71	4.73	4.72	4.72	4.72	4.73	4.73	4.73
Set3 (SL 1:3)	4.71	4.71	4.72	4.71	4.72	4.71	4.70	4.71	4.70	4.70	4.71	4.71
Set4(SL 2:1)	4.71	4.73	4.71	4.71	4.73	4.73	4.73	4.71	4.72	4.73	4.73	4.70
Set5 (SL 3:1)	4.72	4.73	4.71	4.72	4.72	4.72	4.72	4.71	4.72	4.73	4.73	4.72
Average	4.71	4.72	4.72	4.71	4.71	4.72	4.72	4.72	4.71	4.72	4.72	4.72

Not significant

Table 24.4 : The interaction effect of sources of milk, temperature, fat and starter culture on lactose content (%) of yoghurt

Starter Culture	Sources of milk x Temperature x Fat											
	M_1 (Cow milk)						M_2 (Buffalo milk)					
	T_1 (39°C)			T_2 (42°C)			T_1 (39°C)			T_2 (42°C)		
	F_1 (4%)	F_2 (5%)	F_3 (6%)	F_1 (4%)	F_2 (5%)	F_3 (6%)	F_1 (4%)	F_2 (5%)	F_3 (6%)	F_1 (4%)	F_2 (5%)	F_3 (6%)
Set1 (SL 1:1)	5.20	5.17	5.17	5.03	5.10	5.07	5.40	5.37	5.30	5.12	5.20	5.17
Set2 (SL 1:2)	5.37	5.35	5.37	5.27	5.32	5.23	5.57	5.55	5.48	5.37	5.42	5.33
Set3 (SL 1:3)	5.50	5.52	5.50	5.50	5.49	5.40	5.73	5.72	5.62	5.60	5.59	5.50
Set4 (SL 2:1)	5.13	5.14	5.10	4.97	5.05	5.00	5.33	5.34	5.20	5.07	5.15	5.10
Set5 (SL 3:1)	5.00	5.00	4.97	4.88	4.95	4.90	5.13	5.20	5.07	4.98	5.05	4.97
Average	5.24	5.24	5.22	5.13	5.18	5.12	5.43	5.44	5.33	5.23	5.28	5.21

Not significant

Table 24.5 : The interaction effect of sources of milk, temperature, fat and starter culture on ash content (%) of yoghurt

Starter Culture	Sources of milk x Temperature x Fat											
	M_1 (Cow milk)						M_2 (Buffalo milk)					
	T_1 (39°C)			T_2 (42°C)			T_1 (39°C)			T_2 (42°C)		
	F_1 (4%)	F_2 (5%)	F_3 (6%)	F_1 (4%)	F_2 (5%)	F_3 (6%)	F_1 (4%)	F_2 (5%)	F_3 (6%)	F_1 (4%)	F_2 (5%)	F_3 (6%)
Set1 (SL 1:1)	1.02	1.01	1.00	1.00	1.01	1.02	1.01	1.02	1.00	1.00	1.02	1.01
Set2 (SL 1:2)	1.01	1.02	1.01	1.01	1.01	1.01	1.01	1.01	1.02	1.01	1.01	1.02
Set3 (SL 1:3)	1.01	1.02	1.01	1.01	1.01	1.01	1.01	1.01	1.01	1.01	1.01	1.01
Set4(SL 2:1)	1.03	1.03	1.03	1.02	1.03	1.02	1.03	1.02	1.03	1.03	1.03	1.03
Set5 (SL 3:1)	1.03	1.03	1.02	1.03	1.03	1.02	1.03	1.03	1.03	1.02	1.02	1.02
Average	1.02	1.02	1.01	1.01	1.02	1.02	1.02	1.02	1.02	1.01	1.02	1.02

Not significant

Table 24.6 : The interaction effect of sources of milk, temperature, fat and starter culture on lactic acid content (%) of yoghurt

Starter Culture	Sources of milk x Temperature x Fat											
	M₁ (Cow milk)						M₂ (Buffalo milk)					
	T₁ (39°C)			T₂ (42°C)			T₁ (39°C)			T₂ (42°C)		
	F₁ (4%)	F₂ (5%)	F₃ (6%)	F₁ (4%)	F₂ (5%)	F₃ (6%)	F₁ (4%)	F₂ (5%)	F₃ (6%)	F₁ (4%)	F₂ (5%)	F₃ (6%)
Set1 (SL 1:1)	0.87	0.87	0.88	0.89	0.90	0.90	0.88	0.88	0.88	0.90	0.90	0.91
Set2 (SL 1:2)	0.88	0.88	0.88	0.91	0.91	0.91	0.89	0.89	0.89	0.91	0.91	0.91
Set3 (SL 1:3)	0.89	0.89	0.90	0.93	0.94	0.94	0.90	0.91	0.91	0.94	0.94	0.94
Set4(SL 2:1)	1.05	1.06	1.06	1.09	1.09	1.09	1.06	1.06	1.07	1.10	1.10	1.10
Set5 (SL 3:1)	1.07	1.07	1.08	1.14	1.13	1.14	1.08	1.08	1.09	1.14	1.14	1.15
Average	0.95	0.96	0.96	0.99	0.99	1.00	0.96	0.96	0.97	1.00	1.00	1.00

Not significant

Table 24.7 : The interaction effect of sources of milk, temperature, fat and starter culture on pH content (%) of yoghurt

Starter Culture	Sources of milk x Temperature x Fat											
	M₁ (Cow milk)						M₂ (Buffalo milk)					
	T₁ (39°C)			T₂ (42°C)			T₁ (39°C)			T₂ (42°C)		
	F₁ (4%)	F₂ (5%)	F₃ (6%)	F₁ (4%)	F₂ (5%)	F₃ (6%)	F₁ (4%)	F₂ (5%)	F₃ (6%)	F₁ (4%)	F₂ (5%)	F₃ (6%)
Set1 (SL 1:1)	4.670	4.66	4.69	4.61	4.60	4.60	4.67	4.66	4.65	4.60	4.60	4.59
Set2 (SL 1:2)	4.67	4.63	4.62	4.59	4.58	4.58	4.62	4.62	4.62	4.58	4.58	4.58
Set3 (SL 1:3)	4.61	4.65	4.61	4.57	4.56	4.56	4.61	4.60	4.59	4.56	4.56	4.56
Set4(SL 2:1)	4.50	4.48	4.48	4.48	4.46	4.46	4.50	4.50	4.47	4.46	4.46	4.45
Set5 (SL 3:1)	4.47	4.47	4.46	4.40	4.42	4.41	4.46	4.46	4.46	4.41	4.41	4.40
Average	4.59	4.58	4.57	4.53	4.53	4.52	4.57	4.57	4.56	4.52	4.52	4.52

Not significant

Table 24.8 : The interaction effect of sources of milk, temperature, SNF and starter culture on fat content (%) of yoghurt

Starter Culture	Sources of milk x Temperature x Fat											
	M_1 (Cow milk)						M_2 (Buffalo milk)					
	T_1 (39°C)			T_2 (42°C)			T_1 (39°C)			T_2 (42°C)		
	S_1 (10%)	S_2 (11%)	S_3 (12%)	S_1 (10%)	S_2 (11%)	S_3 (12%)	S_1 (10%)	S_2 (11%)	S_3 (12%)	S_1 (10%)	S_2 (11%)	S_3 (12%)
Set1 (SL 1:1)	5.05	5.03	5.03	5.01	5.05	5.03	5.01	5.02	5.03	5.03	5.01	5.03
Set2 (SL 1:2)	5.01	5.00	5.00	5.01	5.01	5.00	5.01	5.01	5.00	5.01	5.00	5.02
Set3 (SL 1:3)	5.02	5.03	5.00	5.02	5.03	5.02	5.02	5.03	5.02	5.02	5.03	5.00
Set4(SL 2:1)	5.02	5.04	5.01	5.02	5.04	5.04	5.03	5.04	5.04	5.02	5.04	5.03
Set5 (SL 3:1)	5.02	5.01	5.01	5.02	5.01	5.01	5.00	5.01	5.01	5.02	5.02	5.01
Average	5.02	5.02	5.01	5.01	5.03	5.02	5.01	5.02	5.02	5.02	5.02	5.02

Not significant

Table 24.9 : The interaction effect of sources of milk, temperature, SNF and starter culture on fat content (%) of yoghurt

Starter Culture	Sources of milk x Temperature x Fat											
	M_1 (Cow milk)						M_2 (Buffalo milk)					
	T_1 (39°C)			T_2 (42°C)			T_1 (39°C)			T_2 (42°C)		
	S_1 (10%)	S_2 (11%)	S_3 (12%)	S_1 (10%)	S_2 (11%)	S_3 (12%)	S_1 (10%)	S_2 (11%)	S_3 (12%)	S_1 (10%)	S_2 (11%)	S_3 (12%)
Set1 (SL 1:1)	4.30	4.65	5.18	4.30	4.62	5.18	4.30	4.67	5.18	4.30	4.67	5.18
Set2 (SL 1:2)	4.28	4.60	5.20	4.29	4.68	5.20	4.28	4.70	5.19	4.28	4.70	5.20
Set3 (SL 1:3)	4.30	4.67	5.19	4.30	4.65	5.19	4.30	4.62	5.19	4.30	4.63	5.19
Set4(SL 2:1)	4.29	4.67	5.20	4.28	4.68	5.20	4.29	4.67	5.20	4.29	4.67	5.20
Set5 (SL 3:1)	4.29	4.68	5.18	4.29	4.70	5.17	4.29	4.68	5.18	4.29	4.70	5.19
Average	4.29	4.67	5.19	4.29	4.67	5.19	4.29	4.67	5.19	4.29	4.67	5.19

Not significant

Table 25.0 : The interaction effects of sources of milk, temperature, SNF and starter culture on lactose (%) of yoghurt

Starter Culture	Sources of milk x Temperature x Fat											
	M$_1$ (Cow milk)						M$_2$ (Buffalo milk)					
	T$_1$ (39°C)			T$_2$ (42°C)			T$_1$ (39°C)			T$_2$ (42°C)		
	S$_1$ 10%	S$_2$ 11%	S$_3$ 12%	S$_1$ 10%	S$_2$ 11%	S$_3$ 12%	S$_1$ 10%	S$_2$ 11%	S$_3$ 12%	S$_1$ 10%	S$_2$ 11%	S$_3$ 12%
Set1 (SL 1:1)	4.77	5.10	5.67	4.67	5.03	5.50	4.97	5.27	5.83	4.75	5.13	5.60
Set2 (SL 1:2)	4.90	5.28	5.90	4.78	5.23	5.80	5.08	5.45	6.07	4.88	5.33	5.90
Set3 (SL 1:3)	5.02	5.50	6.00	4.97	5.46	5.97	5.23	5.67	6.17	5.07	5.56	6.07
Set4(SL 2:1)	4.68	5.21	5.48	4.57	5.07	5.38	4.85	5.38	5.65	4.67	5.17	5.48
Set5 (SL 3:1)	4.57	5.00	5.40	4.47	4.98	5.28	4.70	5.17	5.53	4.57	5.08	5.35
Average	4.79	5.22	5.69	4.69	5.15	5.59	4.97	5.39	5.85	4.79	5.25	5.68

Not significant

Table 25.1 : The interaction effects of sources of milk, temperature, SNF and starter culture on lactose content (%) of yoghurt

Starter Culture	Sources of milk x Temperature x Fat											
	M$_1$ (Cow milk)						M$_2$ (Buffalo milk)					
	T$_1$ (39°C)			T$_2$ (42°C)			T$_1$ (39°C)			T$_2$ (42°C)		
	S$_1$ 10%	S$_2$ 11%	S$_3$ 12%	S$_1$ 10%	S$_2$ 11%	S$_3$ 12%	S$_1$ 10%	S$_2$ 11%	S$_3$ 12%	S$_1$ (10%	S$_2$ 11%	S$_3$ 12%
Set1 (SL 1:1)	0.88	0.96	1.19	0.87	0.97	1.19	0.87	0.97	1.20	0.88	0.97	1.19
Set2 (SL 1:2)	0.88	0.97	1.19	0.88	0.96	1.19	0.88	0.96	1.20	0.88	0.97	1.19
Set3 (SL 1:3)	0.87	0.97	1.02	0.87	0.97	1.19	0.87	0.97	1.20	0.87	0.97	1.19
Set4(SL 2:1)	0.89	0.97	1.22	0.88	0.97	1.23	0.88	0.97	1.22	0.89	0.97	1.22
Set5 (SL 3:1)	0.89	0.98	1.21	0.88	0.98	1.21	0.89	0.98	1.22	0.88	0.98	1.20
Average	0.88	0.97	1.20	0.88	0.97	1.20	0.88	0.97	1.21	0.88	0.97	1.20

Not significant

Table 25.2 : The interaction effect of sources of milk, temperature, SNF and starter culture on lactic acid content (%) of yoghurt

Starter Culture	Sources of milk x Temperature x Fat											
	M_1 (Cow milk)						M_2 (Buffalo milk)					
	T_1 (39°C)			T_2 (42°C)			T_1 (39°C)			T_2 (42°C)		
	S_1 10%	S_2 11%	S_3 12%	S_1 10%	S_2 11%	S_3 12%	S_1 10%	S_2 11%	S_3 12%	S_1 10%	S_2 11%	S_3 12%
Set1 (SL 1:1)	0.85	0.87	0.90	0.87	0.88	0.94	0.86	0.88	0.91	0.88	0.89	0.95
Set2 (SL 1:2)	0.86	0.88	0.91	0.88	0.89	0.96	0.86	0.88	0.92	0.88	0.90	0.96
Set3 (SL 1:3)	0.86	0.90	0.92	0.88	0.95	0.97	0.87	0.91	0.94	0.89	0.96	0.98
Set4(SL 2:1)	0.99	1.08	1.01	1.03	1.12	1.13	1.00	1.09	1.01	1.04	1.13	1.13
Set5 (SL 3:1)	1.00	1.10	1.12	1.14	1.13	1.15	1.01	1.01	1.14	1.12	1.15	1.16
Average	0.91	0.96	0.99	0.96	0.99	1.03	0.92	0.97	1.00	0.96	1.00	1.04

Not significant

Table 25.3 : The interaction effect of sources of milk, temperature, SNF and starter culture on pH of yoghurt

Starter Culture	Sources of milk x Temperature x Fat											
	M_1 (Cow milk)						M_2 (Buffalo milk)					
	T_1 (39°C)			T_2 (42°C)			T_1 (39°C)			T_2 (42°C)		
	S_1 10%	S_2 11%	S_3 12%	S_1 10%	S_2 11%	S_3 12%	S_1 10%	S_2 11%	S_3 12%	S_1 10%	S_2 11%	S_3 12%
Set1 (SL 1:1)	4.80	4.66	4.59	4.63	4.61	4.56	4.78	4.61	4.58	4.62	4.61	4.56
Set2 (SL 1:2)	4.73	4.61	4.58	4.62	4.59	4.55	4.69	4.60	4.57	4.60	4.59	4.55
Set3 (SL 1:3)	4.67	4.63	4.57	4.60	4.55	4.54	4.65	4.58	4.56	4.60	4.55	4.54
Set4(SL 2:1)	4.54	4.45	4.46	4.52	4.47	4.42	4.54	4.45	4.48	4.51	4.43	4.43
Set5 (SL 3:1)	4.53	4.44	4.43	4.42	4.42	4.39	4.53	4.44	4.42	4.43	4.41	4.38
Average	4.65	4.56	4.53	4.56	4.53	4.49	4.64	4.54	4.52	4.55	4.52	4.49

Not significant

Table 25.4 : The interaction effect of temperature, fat, SNF and starter culture on fat content (%) of yoghurt

Starter culture	Temperature x Fat x SNF																	
	T₁ (39°C)									T₂ (42°C)								
	F₁ (4%)			F₂ (5%)			F₃ (6%)			F₁ (4%)			F₂ (5%)			F₃ (6%)		
	S1 (10%)	S2 (11%)	S3 (12%)	S1 (10%)	S2 (11%)	S3 (12%)	S1 (10%)	S2 (11%)	S3 (12%)	S1 (10%)	S2 (11%)	S3 (12%)	S1 (10%)	S2 (11%)	S3 (12%)	S1 (10%)	S2 (11%)	S3 (12%)
Set1 (SL 1:1)	4.06	4.05	4.05	5.01	5.00	5.02	6.03	6.03	6.02	4.02	4.06	4.10	5.01	5.00	5.00	6.03	6.03	6.00
Set2 (SL 1:2)	4.00	4.02	4.00	5.00	5.00	5.00	6.03	6.01	6.00	4.00	4.02	4.00	5.00	5.00	5.01	6.03	6.01	6.02
Set3 (SL 1:3)	4.05	4.00	4.00	5.00	5.00	5.03	6.00	6.10	6.00	4.05	4.00	4.00	5.00	5.00	5.03	6.00	6.10	6.00
Set4 (SL 2:1)	4.00	4.08	4.01	5.05	5.01	5.04	6.02	6.04	6.03	4.00	4.08	4.04	5.05	5.01	5.04	6.00	6.04	6.03
Set5 (SL 3:1)	4.00	4.03	4.00	5.04	5.00	5.02	6.00	6.00	6.00	4.00	4.03	4.00	5.07	5.02	5.02	6.00	6.00	6.00
Average	4.02	4.04	4.01	5.02	5.00	5.02	6.02	6.04	6.01	4.01	4.04	4.03	5.03	5.01	5.02	6.01	6.04	6.01

Not significant

Table 25.5 : The interaction effect of temperature, fat, SNF and starter culture on protein content (%) of yoghurt.

Temperature x Fat x SNF

Starter culture	T₁ F₁(4%) S1 (10%)	T₁ F₁(4%) S2 (11%)	T₁ F₁(4%) S3 (12%)	T₁ F₂(5%) S1 (10%)	T₁ F₂(5%) S2 (11%)	T₁ F₂(5%) S3 (12%)	T₁ F₃(6%) S1 (10%)	T₁ F₃(6%) S2 (11%)	T₁ F₃(6%) S3 (12%)	T₂ F₁(4%) S1 (10%)	T₂ F₁(4%) S2 (11%)	T₂ F₁(4%) S3 (12%)	T₂ F₂(5%) S1 (10%)	T₂ F₂(5%) S2 (11%)	T₂ F₂(5%) S3 (12%)	T₂ F₃(6%) S1 (10%)	T₂ F₃(6%) S2 (11%)	T₂ F₃(6%) S3 (12%)
Set1 (SL 1:1)	4.30	4.63	5.18	4.30	4.70	5.18	4.30	4.65	5.18	4.30	4.60	5.18	4.30	4.65	5.18	4.29	4.68	5.19
Set2 (SL 1:2)	4.28	4.70	5.20	4.28	4.70	5.20	4.28	4.70	5.19	4.29	4.70	5.20	4.29	4.68	5.20	4.29	4.70	5.20
Set3 (SL 1:3)	4.03	4.63	5.20	4.30	4.65	5.19	4.30	4.65	5.19	4.30	4.63	5.20	4.30	4.65	5.20	4.30	4.65	5.19
Set4 (SL 2:1)	4.29	4.68	5.20	4.29	4.68	5.20	4.29	4.65	5.20	4.028	4.68	5.20	4.29	4.70	5.20	4.29	4.65	5.20
Set5 (SL 3:1)	4.29	4.70	5.17	4.30	4.68	5.19	4.30	4.68	5.19	4.30	4.70	5.18	4.29	4.70	53.18	4.30	4.70	5.18
Average	4.29	4.67	5.19	4.29	4.68	5.19	4.29	4.67	5.19	4.29	4.66	5.19	4.29	4.68	5.19	4.29	4.68	5.19

Not significant

Table 25.6 : The interaction effect of temperature, fat, SNF and starter culture on lactose content (%) of yoghurt

Temperature x Fat x SNF

Starter culture	T₁ F₁(4%) S1 (10%)	T₁ F₁(4%) S2 (11%)	T₁ F₁(4%) S3 (12%)	T₁ F₂(5%) S1 (10%)	T₁ F₂(5%) S2 (11%)	T₁ F₂(5%) S3 (12%)	T₁ F₃(6%) S1 (10%)	T₁ F₃(6%) S2 (11%)	T₁ F₃(6%) S3 (12%)	T₂ F₁(4%) S1 (10%)	T₂ F₁(4%) S2 (11%)	T₂ F₁(4%) S3 (12%)	T₂ F₂(5%) S1 (10%)	T₂ F₂(5%) S2 (11%)	T₂ F₂(5%) S3 (12%)	T₂ F₃(6%) S1 (10%)	T₂ F₃(6%) S2 (11%)	T₂ F₃(6%) S3 (12%)
Set1 (SL 1:1)	4.90	5.20	5.80	4.92	5.20	5.70	4.80	5.15	5.75	4.73	5.05	5.45	4.75	5.05	5.65	4.65	5.15	5.55
Set2 (SL 1:2)	5.00	5.40	6.00	5.00	5.35	6.00	4.98	5.35	5.95	4.85	5.25	5.85	4.90	5.35	5.85	4.75	5.25	5.85
Set3 (SL 1:3)	5.15	5.60	6.10	5.15	5.60	6.10	5.08	5.55	6.05	5.05	5.55	6.05	5.05	5.52	6.05	4.95	5.45	5.95
Set4 (SL 2:1)	4.80	5.30	5.60	4.85	5.33	5.55	4.65	5.25	5.55	4.65	5.05	5.35	4.65	5.15	5.50	4.55	5.15	5.45
Set5 (SL 3:1)	4.65	5.10	5.45	4.70	5.10	5.50	4.55	5.05	5.45	4.55	5.00	5.25	4.55	5.05	5.40	4.45	5.05	5.30
Average	4.90	5.32	5.79	4.92	5.32	5.77	4.81	5.27	5.75	4.77	5.18	5.59	4.78	5.22	5.69	4.67	5.21	5.62

Not significant

Table 25.7 : The interaction effect of temperature, fat, SNF and starter culture on ash content (%) of yoghurt

Starter culture	Temperature x Fat x SNF																	
	T_1 (39°C)									T_2 (42°C)								
	F_1 (4%)			F_2 (5%)			F_3 (6%)			F_1 (4%)			F_2 (5%)			F_3 (6%)		
	S1 (10%)	S2 (11%)	S3 (12%)	S1 (10%)	S2 (11%)	S3 (12%)	S1 (10%)	S2 (11%)	S3 (12%)	S1 (10%)	S2 (11%)	S3 (12%)	S1 (10%)	S2 (11%)	S3 (12%)	S1 (10%)	S2 (11%)	S3 (12%)
Set1 (SL 1:1)	0.88	0.97	1.20	0.88	0.97	1.21	0.87	0.97	1.18	0.87	0.97	1.18	0.88	0.97	1.19	0.88	0.97	1.20
Set2 (SL 1:2)	0.88	0.96	1.20	0.88	0.97	1.20	0.88	0.97	1.20	0.88	0.97	1.19	0.88	0.97	1.19	0.88	0.97	1.20
Set3 (SL 1:3)	0.88	0.97	1.19	0.87	0.96	1.22	0.88	0.98	1.19	0.87	0.98	1.19	0.88	0.98	1.19	0.87	0.96	1.20
Set4 (SL 2:1)	0.89	0.98	1.22	0.88	0.97	1.22	0.89	0.97	1.23	0.89	0.97	1.22	0.89	0.98	1.23	0.88	0.97	1.23
Set5 (SL 3:1)	0.90	0.98	1.21	0.89	0.98	1.22	0.88	0.98	1.21	0.88	0.98	1.21	0.88	0.98	1.21	0.89	0.98	1.20
Average	0.88	0.97	1.20	0.89	0.97	1.21	0.88	0.97	1.20	0.88	0.97	1.20	0.88	0.98	1.20	0.88	0.97	1.20

Not significant

Table 25.8 : The interaction effect of temperature, fat, SNF and culture on lactic acid content (%) of yoghurt

Starter culture	Temperature x Fat x SNF																	
	T_1 (39°C)									T_2 (42°C)								
	F_1 (4%)			F_2 (5%)			F_3 (6%)			F_1 (4%)			F_2 (5%)			F_3 (6%)		
	S1 (10%)	S2 (11%)	S3 (12%)	S1 (10%)	S2 (11%)	S3 (12%)	S1 (10%)	S2 (11%)	S3 (12%)	S1 (10%)	S2 (11%)	S3 (12%)	S1 (10%)	S2 (11%)	S3 (12%)	S1 (10%)	S2 (11%)	S3 (12%)
Set1 (SL 1:1)	0.85	0.87	0.90	0.85	0.88	0.91	0.85	0.88	0.91	0.87	0.88	0.94	0.87	0.88	0.95	0.87	0.88	0.95
Set2 (SL 1:2)	0.86	0.88	0.92	0.86	0.88	0.92	0.86	0.88	0.92	0.88	0.90	0.95	0.88	0.89	0.96	0.88	0.89	0.96
Set3 (SL 1:3)	0.86	0.90	0.93	0.86	0.91	0.93	0.87	0.91	0.93	0.88	0.95	0.97	0.89	0.96	0.98	0.89	0.96	0.98
Set4 (SL 2:1)	0.99	1.08	1.10	0.99	1.09	1.10	1.00	1.09	1.10	1.04	1.12	1.12	1.03	1.13	1.13	1.03	1.13	1.14
Set5 (SL 3:1)	1.00	1.10	1.12	1.00	1.10	1.13	1.02	1.10	1.13	1.13	1.14	1.14	1.12	1.14	1.16	1.12	1.15	1.17
Average	0.91	0.96	0.99	0.91	0.97	1.00	0.92	0.97	1.00	0.96	1.00	1.03	0.96	1.00	1.03	0.96	1.00	1.04

Not significant

Table 25.9 : The interaction effect of temperature, fat, SNF and starter culture on pH of yoghurt

Starter culture	T₁ (39°C) F₁(4%) S1 (10%)	T₁ (39°C) F₁(4%) S2 (11%)	T₁ (39°C) F₁(4%) S3 (12%)	T₁ (39°C) F₂(5%) S1 (10%)	T₁ (39°C) F₂(5%) S2 (11%)	T₁ (39°C) F₂(5%) S3 (12%)	T₁ (39°C) F₃(6%) S1 (10%)	T₁ (39°C) F₃(6%) S2 (11%)	T₁ (39°C) F₃(6%) S3 (12%)	T₂ (42°C) F₁(4%) S1 (10%)	T₂ (42°C) F₁(4%) S2 (11%)	T₂ (42°C) F₁(4%) S3 (12%)	T₂ (42°C) F₂(5%) S1 (10%)	T₂ (42°C) F₂(5%) S2 (11%)	T₂ (42°C) F₂(5%) S3 (12%)	T₂ (42°C) F₃(6%) S1 (10%)	T₂ (42°C) F₃(6%) S2 (11%)	T₂ (42°C) F₃(6%) S3 (12%)
Set1 (SL 1:1)	4.83	4.63	4.59	4.78	4.62	4.58	4.77	4.65	4.59	4.64	4.61	4.56	4.62	4.61	4.56	4.62	4.61	4.56
Set2 (SL 1:2)	4.75	4.61	4.58	4.70	4.60	4.58	4.68	4.61	4.58	4.62	4.58	4.56	4.61	4.59	4.55	4.61	4.59	4.55
Set3 (SL 1:3)	4.67	4.60	4.57	4.67	4.64	4.57	4.66	4.58	4.57	4.60	4.56	4.54	4.60	4.55	4.54	4.60	4.55	4.54
Set4 (SL 2:1)	4.54	4.46	4.50	4.53	4.46	4.47	4.54	4.45	4.44	4.51	4.48	4.43	4.52	4.44	4.43	4.52	4.43	4.42
Set5 (SL 3:1)	4.52	4.44	4.44	4.53	4.44	4.43	4.53	4.43	4.43	4.41	4.42	4.41	4.44	4.42	4.39	4.43	4.41	4.37
Average	4.66	4.55	4.53	4.64	4.55	4.52	4.63	4.54	4.52	4.56	4.53	4.50	4.56	4.52	4.49	4.55	4.52	4.49

Not significant

Table 26.0 : The interaction effect of fat, sources of milk, SNF and starter culture on fat content (%) of yoghurt

Starter culture	M₁ (Cow milk) F₁(4%) S1 (10%)	M₁ (Cow milk) F₁(4%) S2 (11%)	M₁ (Cow milk) F₁(4%) S3 (12%)	M₁ (Cow milk) F₂(5%) S1 (10%)	M₁ (Cow milk) F₂(5%) S2 (11%)	M₁ (Cow milk) F₂(5%) S3 (12%)	M₁ (Cow milk) F₃(6%) S1 (10%)	M₁ (Cow milk) F₃(6%) S2 (11%)	M₁ (Cow milk) F₃(6%) S3 (12%)	M₂ (Buffalo milk) F₁(4%) S1 (10%)	M₂ (Buffalo milk) F₁(4%) S2 (11%)	M₂ (Buffalo milk) F₁(4%) S3 (12%)	M₂ (Buffalo milk) F₂(5%) S1 (10%)	M₂ (Buffalo milk) F₂(5%) S2 (11%)	M₂ (Buffalo milk) F₂(5%) S3 (12%)	M₂ (Buffalo milk) F₃(6%) S1 (10%)	M₂ (Buffalo milk) F₃(6%) S2 (11%)	M₂ (Buffalo milk) F₃(6%) S3 (12%)
Set1 (SL 1:1)	4.05	4.10	4.10	5.01	5.00	5.00	6.03	6.00	6.00	4.03	4.01	4.05	5.01	5.00	5.02	6.03	6.03	6.02
Set2 (SL 1:2)	4.00	4.02	4.00	5.00	5.00	5.00	6.03	6.01	6.00	4.00	4.02	4.00	5.00	5.00	5.01	6.03	6.01	6.02
Set3 (SL 1:3)	4.05	4.00	4.00	5.00	5.00	5.03	6.00	6.10	6.00	4.05	4.00	4.00	5.00	5.00	5.03	6.00	6.10	6.00
Set4 (SL 2:1)	4.00	4.08	4.01	5.05	5.01	5.04	6.00	6.04	6.03	4.00	4.08	4.04	5.05	5.01	5.04	6.02	6.04	6.03
Set5 (SL 3:1)	4.00	4.03	4.00	5.07	5.00	5.02	6.00	6.00	6.00	4.00	4.03	4.00	5.04	5.02	5.02	6.00	6.00	6.00
Average	4.02	4.05	4.02	5.03	5.00	5.02	6.01	6.04	6.01	4.02	4.03	4.02	5.02	5.01	5.02	6.02	6.04	6.01

Not significant

Table 26.1 : The interaction effect of fat, sources of milk, SNF and starter culture on protein (%) of yoghurt

Fat x Sources of milk x SNF

Starter culture	M₁ (Cow milk)									M₂ (Buffalo milk)								
	F₁ (4%)			F₂ (5%)			F₃ (6%)			F₁ (4%)			F₂ (5%)			F₃ (6%)		
	S1 (10%)	S2 (11%)	S3 (12%)	S1 (10%)	S2 (11%)	S3 (12%)	S1 (10%)	S2 (11%)	S3 (12%)	S1 (10%)	S2 (11%)	S3 (12%)	S1 (10%)	S2 (11%)	S3 (12%)	S1 (10%)	S2 (11%)	S3 (12%)
Set1 (SL 1:1)	4.30	4.60	5.18	4.30	4.65	5.18	4.30	4.65	5.18	4.30	4.63	5.18	4.30	4.70	5.18	4.30	4.68	5.19
Set2 (SL 1:2)	4.29	4.70	5.20	4.29	4.68	5.20	4.29	4.70	5.20	4.25	4.70	5.20	4.28	4.70	5.20	4.29	4.70	5.20
Set3 (SL 1:3)	4.30	4.65	5.19	4.30	4.65	5.20	4.30	4.68	5.19	4.30	4.60	5.20	4.30	4.65	5.19	4.30	4.63	5.19
Set4 (SL 2:1)	4.28	4.65	5.20	4.29	4.70	5.20	4.28	4.68	5.20	4.29	4.70	5.20	4.29	4.68	5.20	4.30	4.63	5.20
Set5 (SL 3:1)	4.29	4.70	5.17	4.29	4.70	5.18	4.30	4.68	5.18	4.30	4.70	5.18	4.30	4.68	5.19	4.20	4.70	5.18
Average	4.29	4.66	5.19	4.29	4.68	5.19	4.29	4.68	5.19	4.29	4.67	5.19	4.29	4.68	5.19	4.20	4.67	5.19

Not significant

Table 26.2 : The interaction effect of fat, sources of milk, SNF and starter culture on lactose content (%) of yoghurt

Fat x Sources of milk x SNF

Starter culture	M₁ (Cow milk)									M₂ (Buffalo milk)								
	F₁ (4%)			F₂ (5%)			F₃ (6%)			F₁ (4%)			F₂ (5%)			F₃ (6%)		
	S1 (10%)	S2 (11%)	S3 (12%)	S1 (10%)	S2 (11%)	S3 (12%)	S1 (10%)	S2 (11%)	S3 (12%)	S1 (10%)	S2 (11%)	S3 (12%)	S1 (10%)	S2 (11%)	S3 (12%)	S1 (10%)	S2 (11%)	S3 (12%)
Set1 (SL 1:1)	4.75	5.05	5.55	4.76	5.05	5.60	4.65	5.10	5.60	4.88	5.20	5.70	4.91	5.20	5.75	4.80	5.20	5.70
Set2 (SL 1:2)	4.85	5.25	53.85	4.88	5.28	5.85	4.80	5.25	5.85	5.00	5.40	6.00	5.03	5.43	6.00	4.93	5.35	5.95
Set3 (SL 1:3)	5.00	5.50	6.00	5.03	5.49	6.00	4.95	5.45	5.95	5.20	5.65	6.15	5.18	5.64	6.15	5.08	5.55	6.05
Set4 (SL 2:1)	4.65	5.10	5.40	4.68	5.17	5.45	4.55	5.15	5.45	4.80	5.25	5.55	4.83	5.32	5.60	4.65	5.25	5.55
Set5 (SL 3:1)	4.55	4.98	5.30	4.55	5.00	5.38	4.45	5.15	5.35	4.65	5.13	5.40	4.70	5.15	5.53	4.55	5.10	5.54
Average	4.76	5.18	5.62	4.78	5.20	5.66	4.68	5.00	5.64	4.91	5.33	5.76	4.93	5.35	5.81	4.80	5.29	5.73

Not significant

Table 26.3 : The interaction effect of fat, sources of milk, SNF and starter culture on lactose content (%) of yoghurt

Starter culture	M₁ (Cow milk)									M₂ (Buffalo milk)								
	F₁ (4%)			F₂ (5%)			F₃ (6%)			F₁ (4%)			F₂ (5%)			F₃ (6%)		
	S1 (10%)	S2 (11%)	S3 (12%)	S1 (10%)	S2 (11%)	S3 (12%)	S1 (10%)	S2 (11%)	S3 (12%)	S1 (10%)	S2 (11%)	S3 (12%)	S1 (10%)	S2 (11%)	S3 (12%)	S1 (10%)	S2 (11%)	S3 (12%)
Set1 (SL 1:1)	0.88	0.97	1.19	0.87	0.97	1.19	0.88	0.97	1.20	0.87	0.96	1.19	0.89	0.97	1.21	0.87	0.97	1.18
Set2 (SL 1:2)	0.88	0.97	1.19	0.88	0.98	1.19	0.88	0.96	1.20	0.88	0.96	1.20	0.88	0.96	1.20	0.88	0.98	1.20
Set3 (SL 1:3)	0.88	0.98	1.19	0.87	0.97	1.21	0.87	0.97	1.19	0.87	0.97	1.19	0.88	0.97	1.19	0.87	0.97	1.20
Set4 (SL 2:1)	0.89	0.98	1.21	0.89	0.97	1.23	0.88	0.97	1.23	0.89	0.97	1.22	0.88	0.98	1.22	0.89	0.97	1.23
Set5 (SL 3:1)	0.89	0.98	1.22	0.89	0.98	1.21	0.88	0.98	1.20	0.89	0.98	1.20	0.88	0.98	1.22	0.89	0.98	1.21
Average	0.88	0.98	1.20	0.88	0.97	1.21	0.88	0.97	1.20	0.88	0.97	1.20	0.88	0.97	1.21	0.88	0.97	1.20

Not significant

Table 26.4 : The interaction effect of fat, sources of milk, SNF and starter culture on lactic acid content (%) of yoghurt

Starter culture	M₁ (Cow milk)									M₂ (Buffalo milk)								
	F₁ (4%)			F₂ (5%)			F₃ (6%)			F₁ (4%)			F₂ (5%)			F₃ (6%)		
	S1 (10%)	S2 (11%)	S3 (12%)	S1 (10%)	S2 (11%)	S3 (12%)	S1 (10%)	S2 (11%)	S3 (12%)	S1 (10%)	S2 (11%)	S3 (12%)	S1 (10%)	S2 (11%)	S3 (12%)	S1 (10%)	S2 (11%)	S3 (12%)
Set1 (SL 1:1)	0.86	0.87	0.92	0.86	0.88	0.92	0.86	0.88	0.92	0.86	0.88	0.93	0.87	0.88	0.93	0.87	0.88	0.93
Set2 (SL 1:2)	0.87	0.88	0.93	0.87	0.89	0.93	0.87	0.89	0.94	0.87	0.89	0.94	0.87	0.89	0.94	0.87	0.89	0.94
Set3 (SL 1:3)	0.87	0.92	0.94	0.87	0.93	0.95	0.87	0.93	0.95	0.88	0.93	0.96	0.88	0.94	0.96	0.88	0.94	0.96
Set4 (SL 2:1)	1.01	1.09	1.11	1.01	1.10	1.12	1.01	1.10	1.12	1.01	1.11	1.11	1.01	1.11	1.12	1.02	1.11	1.12
Set5 (SL 3:1)	1.08	1.11	1.12	1.06	1.12	1.13	1.07	1.14	1.17	1.05	1.13	1.14	1.06	1.13	1.15	1.07	1.13	1.16
Average	0.94	0.98	1.01	0.93	0.98	1.01	0.94	0.98	1.01	0.93	0.99	1.01	0.94	0.99	1.02	0.94	0.99	1.02

Not significant

Table 26.5 : The interaction effect of fat, sources of milk, SNF and starter culture on pH of yoghurt

Starter culture	Fat x Sources of milk x SNF																	
	M_1 (Cow milk)									M_2 (Buffalo milk)								
	F_1 (4%)			F_2 (5%)			F_3 (6%)			F_1 (4%)			F_2 (5%)			F_3 (6%)		
	S1 (10%)	S2 (11%)	S3 (12%)	S1 (10%)	S2 (11%)	S3 (12%)	S1 (10%)	S2 (11%)	S3 (12%)	S1 (10%)	S2 (11%)	S3 (12%)	S1 (10%)	S2 (11%)	S3 (12%)	S1 (10%)	S2 (11%)	S3 (12%)
Set1 (SL 1:1)	4.76	4.63	4.58	4.70	4.62	4.57	4.70	4.66	4.58	4.71	4.62	4.57	4.70	4.61	4.57	4.69	4.60	4.57
Set2 (SL 1:2)	4.72	4.60	4.57	4.66	4.60	4.57	4.65	4.60	4.57	4.66	4.59	4.57	4.65	4.60	4.56	4.64	4.60	4.56
Set3 (SL 1:3)	4.64	4.58	4.56	4.64	4.63	4.56	4.63	4.57	4.56	4.63	4.57	4.56	4.63	4.57	4.55	4.63	4.56	4.55
Set4 (SL 2:1)	4.53	4.49	4.46	4.53	4.45	4.44	4.53	4.45	4.43	4.53	4.45	4.47	4.53	4.44	4.47	4.52	4.43	4.43
Set5 (SL 3:1)	4.45	4.43	4.43	4.49	4.44	4.41	4.48	4.42	4.41	4.48	4.43	4.42	4.49	4.43	4.40	4.48	4.42	4.39
Average	4.62	4.54	4.52	4.60	4.55	4.51	4.60	4.54	4.51	4.60	4.53	4.52	4.60	4.53	4.51	4.59	4.52	4.50

Not significant

Table 26.6 : The interaction effect of temperature, sources of milk, fat, SNF and starter culture on fat content (%) of yoghurt

Temperature x Sources of milk x Fat x SNF
M₁ (Cow milk)

Starter culture	T₁ (39°C)									T₂ (42°C)								
	F₁ (4%)			F₂ (5%)			F₃ (6%)			F₁ (4%)			F₂ (5%)			F₃ (6%)		
	S1 (10%)	S2 (11%)	S3 (12%)	S1 (10%)	S2 (11%)	S3 (12%)	S1 (10%)	S2 (11%)	S3 (12%)	S1 (10%)	S2 (11%)	S3 (12%)	S1 (10%)	S2 (11%)	S3 (12%)	S1 (10%)	S2 (11%)	S3 (12%)
Set1 (SL 1:1)	4.10	4.10	4.10	5.00	5.00	5.00	6.06	6.00	6.00	4.00	4.10	4.10	5.02	5.00	5.00	6.00	6.06	6.0
Set2 (SL 1:2)	4.00	4.00	4.00	5.00	5.00	5.00	6.03	6.01	6.00	4.00	4.03	4.00	5.00	5.00	5.00	6.03	6.01	6.00
Set3 (SL 1:3)	4.05	4.00	4.00	5.00	5.00	5.00	6.00	6.10	6.00	4.05	4.00	4.00	5.00	5.00	5.06	6.00	6.10	6.00
Set4 (SL 2:1)	4.00	4.08	4.00	5.05	5.00	5.04	6.00	6.04	6.00	4.00	4.08	4.02	5.05	5.01	5.04	6.00	6.04	6.05
Set5 (SL 3:1)	4.00	4.03	4.00	5.00	5.00	5.02	6.00	6.00	6.00	4.00	4.03	4.00	5.07	5.00	5.02	6.00	6.00	6.00
Average	4.03	4.04	4.02	5.02	5.00	5.01	6.02	6.03	6.00	4.01	4.29	4.02	5.03	5.00	5.02	6.01	6.04	6.01

Temperature x Sources of milk x Fat x SNF
M₂ (Buffalo milk)

Starter culture	T₁ (39°C)									T₂ (42°C)								
	F₁ (4%)			F₂ (5%)			F₃ (6%)			F₁ (4%)			F₂ (5%)			F₃ (6%)		
	S1 (10%)	S2 (11%)	S3 (12%)	S1 (10%)	S2 (11%)	S3 (12%)	S1 (10%)	S2 (11%)	S3 (12%)	S1 (10%)	S2 (11%)	S3 (12%)	S1 (10%)	S2 (11%)	S3 (12%)	S1 (10%)	S2 (11%)	S3 (12%)
Set1 (SL 1:1)	4.02	4.00	4.00	5.02	5.00	5.04	6.00	6.06	6.04	4.03	4.02	4.10	5.00	5.00	5.00	6.06	6.00	6.00
Set2 (SL 1:2)	4.00	4.03	4.00	5.00	5.00	5.00	6.03	6.01	6.00	4.00	4.00	4.00	5.00	5.00	5.02	6.03	6.01	6.04
Set3 (SL 1:3)	4.05	4.00	4.00	5.00	5.00	5.06	6.00	6.10	6.00	4.05	4.00	4.00	5.00	5.00	5.00	6.00	6.10	6.00
Set4 (SL 2:1)	4.00	4.08	4.02	5.05	5.01	5.04	6.03	6.04	6.05	4.00	4.08	4.06	5.05	5.00	5.04	6.00	6.04	6.00
Set5 (SL 3:1)	4.00	4.03	4.00	5.00	5.00	5.02	6.00	6.00	6.00	4.00	4.03	4.00	5.07	5.04	5.02	6.00	6.00	6.00
Average	4.01	4.03	4.00	5.01	5.00	5.03	6.01	6.04	6.02	4.02	4.03	4.03	5.02	5.01	5.02	6.02	6.03	6.01

Not significant

Table 26.7 : The interaction effect of temperature, sources of milk, fat, SNF and starter culture on protein content (%) of yoghurt

Temperature x Sources of milk x Fat x SNF — M₁ (Cow milk)

Starter culture	T₁ (39°C)									T₂ (42°C)								
	F₁ (4%)			F₂ (5%)			F₃ (6%)			F₁ (4%)			F₂ (5%)			F₃ (6%)		
	S1 (10%)	S2 (11%)	S3 (12%)	S1 (10%)	S2 (11%)	S3 (12%)	S1 (10%)	S2 (11%)	S3 (12%)	S1 (10%)	S2 (11%)	S3 (12%)	S1 (10%)	S2 (11%)	S3 (12%)	S1 (10%)	S2 (11%)	S3 (12%)
Set1 (SL 1:1)	4.30	4.60	5.18	4.29	4.70	5.18	4.30	4.65	5.18	4.30	4.60	5.18	4.30	4.60	5.18	4.29	4.65	5.18
Set2 (SL 1:2)	4.29	4.70	5.20	4.28	4.70	5.20	4.28	4.70	5.19	4.29	4.70	5.20	4.29	4.65	5.20	4.29	4.70	5.20
Set3 (SL 1:3)	4.30	4.65	5.19	4.30	4.65	5.19	4.29	4.70	5.18	4.30	4.65	5.19	4.30	4.65	5.20	4.30	4.65	5.19
Set4 (SL 2:1)	4.28	4.65	5.20	4.30	4.70	5.20	4.28	4.65	5.20	4.28	4.65	5.20	4.28	4.70	5.20	4.28	4.70	5.20
Set5 (SL 3:1)	4.29	4.70	5.17	4.29	4.70	5.17	4.30	4.65	5.19	4.29	4.70	5.17	4.29	4.70	5.17	4.30	4.70	5.17
Average	4.29	4.66	5.19	4.29	4.69	5.19	4.29	4.67	5.19	4.29	4.66	5.19	4.29	4.66	5.19	4.29	4.68	5.19

Temperature x Sources of milk x Fat x SNF — M₂ (Buffalo milk)

Starter culture	T₁ (39°C)									T₂ (42°C)								
	F₁ (4%)			F₂ (5%)			F₃ (6%)			F₁ (4%)			F₂ (5%)			F₃ (6%)		
	S1 (10%)	S2 (11%)	S3 (12%)	S1 (10%)	S2 (11%)	S3 (12%)	S1 (10%)	S2 (11%)	S3 (12%)	S1 (10%)	S2 (11%)	S3 (12%)	S1 (10%)	S2 (11%)	S3 (12%)	S1 (10%)	S2 (11%)	S3 (12%)
Set1 (SL 1:1)	4.30	4.65	5.18	4.30	4.70	5.18	4.30	4.65	5.18	4.30	4.60	5.18	4.30	4.70	5.17	4.29	4.70	5.19
Set2 (SL 1:2)	4.27	4.70	5.20	4.28	4.70	5.19	4.28	4.70	5.19	4.28	4.70	5.20	4.08	4.70	5.20	4.29	4.70	5.20
Set3 (SL 1:3)	4.30	4.60	5.20	4.29	4.65	5.18	4.29	4.60	5.19	4.30	4.60	5.20	4.30	4.65	5.19	4.30	4.65	5.19
Set4 (SL 2:1)	4.30	4.70	5.19	4.28	4.65	5.20	4.30	4.65	5.20	4.28	4.70	5.20	4.29	4.70	5.20	4.30	4.60	5.20
Set5 (SL 3:1)	4.29	4.70	5.17	4.30	4.65	5.19	4.29	4.70	5.18	4.30	4.70	5.19	4.29	4.70	5.19	4.29	4.70	5.18
Average	4.29	4.67	5.19	4.29	4.67	5.19	4.29	4.66	5.19	4.29	4.66	5.19	4.29	4.69	5.19	4.29	4.67	5.19

Not significant

Table 26.8 : The interaction effect of temperature, sources of milk, fat, SNF and starter culture on lactose content (%) of yoghurt

Temperature x Sources of milk x Fat x SNF

M₁ (Cow milk)

Starter culture	T₁ (39°C)									T₂ (42°C)								
	F₁ (4%)			F₂ (5%)			F₃ (6%)			F₁ (4%)			F₂ (5%)			F₃ (6%)		
	S1 (10%)	S2 (11%)	S3 (12%)	S1 (10%)	S2 (11%)	S3 (12%)	S1 (10%)	S2 (11%)	S3 (12%)	S1 (10%)	S2 (11%)	S3 (12%)	S1 (10%)	S2 (11%)	S3 (12%)	S1 (10%)	S2 (11%)	S3 (12%)
Set1 (SL 1:1)	4.80	5.10	5.70	4.82	5.10	5.60	4.70	5.10	5.70	4.70	5.00	5.40	4.70	5.00	5.60	4.60	5.10	5.50
Set2 (SL 1:2)	4.90	5.30	5.90	4.90	5.25	5.90	4.90	5.30	5.90	4.80	5.20	5.80	4.85	5.30	5.80	4.70	5.20	5.80
Set3 (SL 1:3)	5.00	5.50	6.00	5.05	5.50	6.00	5.00	5.50	6.00	5.00	5.50	6.00	5.00	5.47	6.00	4.90	5.40	5.90
Set4 (SL 2:1)	4.70	5.20	5.50	4.75	5.23	5.45	4.60	5.20	5.50	4.60	5.00	5.30	4.60	5.10	5.45	4.50	5.10	5.40
Set5 (SL 3:1)	4.60	5.00	5.40	4.60	5.00	5.40	4.50	5.00	5.40	4.50	4.95	5.20	4.50	5.00	5.35	4.40	5.00	5.30
Average	4.80	5.22	5.70	4.82	5.22	5.67	4.74	5.22	5.70	4.72	5.13	5.54	4.73	5.17	5.64	4.62	5.16	5.58

Temperature x Sources of milk x Fat x SNF

M₂ (Buffalo milk)

Starter culture	T₁ (39°C)									T₂ (42°C)								
	F₁ (4%)			F₂ (5%)			F₃ (6%)			F₁ (4%)			F₂ (5%)			F₃ (6%)		
	S1 (10%)	S2 (11%)	S3 (12%)	S1 (10%)	S2 (11%)	S3 (12%)	S1 (10%)	S2 (11%)	S3 (12%)	S1 (10%)	S2 (11%)	S3 (12%)	S1 (10%)	S2 (11%)	S3 (12%)	S1 (10%)	S2 (11%)	S3 (12%)
Set1 (SL 1:1)	5.00	5.30	5.90	5.02	5.30	5.80	4.90	5.20	5.80	4.75	5.10	5.50	4.80	5.10	5.70	4.70	5.20	5.60
Set2 (SL 1:2)	5.10	5.50	6.10	5.10	5.45	6.10	5.05	5.40	6.00	4.90	5.30	5.90	4.95	5.40	5.90	4.80	5.30	5.90
Set3 (SL 1:3)	5.30	5.70	6.20	5.25	5.70	6.20	5.15	5.60	6.10	5.10	5.60	6.10	5.10	5.57	6.10	5.00	5.50	6.00
Set4 (SL 2:1)	4.90	5.40	5.70	4.95	5.43	5.65	4.70	5.30	5.60	4.70	5.10	5.40	4.70	5.20	5.55	4.60	5.20	5.50
Set5 (SL 3:1)	4.70	5.20	5.50	4.80	5.20	5.60	4.60	5.10	5.50	4.60	5.05	5.30	4.60	5.10	5.45	4.50	5.10	5.30
Average	5.00	5.42	5.88	5.02	5.40	5.87	4.88	5.32	5.80	4.81	5.23	5.64	4.83	5.27	5.74	4.72	5.26	5.66

Not significant

Table 26.9 : The interaction effects of temperature, sources of milk, fat, SNF and starter culture on ash content (%) of yoghurt

Temperature x Sources of milk x Fat x SNF — M₁ (Cow milk)

Starter culture	T₁ (39°C) F₁ (4%) S1 (10%)	S2 (11%)	S3 (12%)	F₂ (5%) S1 (10%)	S2 (11%)	S3 (12%)	F₃ (6%) S1 (10%)	S2 (11%)	S3 (12%)	T₂ (42°C) F₁ (4%) S1 (10%)	S2 (11%)	S3 (12%)	F₂ (5%) S1 (10%)	S2 (11%)	S3 (12%)	F₃ (6%) S1 (10%)	S2 (11%)	S3 (12%)
Set1 (SL 1:1)	0.89	0.97	1.20	0.87	0.96	1.19	0.87	0.96	1.18	0.86	0.97	1.18	0.87	0.97	1.18	0.88	0.97	1.22
Set2 (SL 1:2)	0.87	0.97	1.19	0.88	0.98	1.20	0.88	0.97	1.19	0.88	0.97	1.18	0.88	0.97	1.18	0.88	0.95	1.20
Set3 (SL 1:3)	0.88	0.98	1.18	0.87	0.96	1.23	0.87	0.98	1.18	0.87	0.98	1.19	0.87	0.98	1.19	0.87	0.96	1.20
Set4 (SL 2:1)	0.89	0.98	1.21	0.89	0.97	1.22	0.89	0.97	1.22	0.88	0.97	1.21	0.89	0.97	1.24	0.86	0.97	1.23
Set5 (SL 3:1)	0.89	0.98	1.22	0.90	0.98	1.20	0.88	0.98	1.20	0.88	0.98	1.22	0.88	0.98	1.22	0.88	0.98	1.20
Average	0.88	0.98	1.20	0.88	0.97	1.21	0.88	0.97	1.19	0.87	0.97	1.20	0.88	0.97	1.20	0.87	0.97	1.21

Temperature x Sources of milk x Fat x SNF — M₂ (Buffalo milk)

Starter culture	T₁ (39°C) F₁ (4%) S1 (10%)	S2 (11%)	S3 (12%)	F₂ (5%) S1 (10%)	S2 (11%)	S3 (12%)	F₃ (6%) S1 (10%)	S2 (11%)	S3 (12%)	T₂ (42°C) F₁ (4%) S1 (10%)	S2 (11%)	S3 (12%)	F₂ (5%) S1 (10%)	S2 (11%)	S3 (12%)	F₃ (6%) S1 (10%)	S2 (11%)	S3 (12%)
Set1 (SL 1:1)	0.87	0.96	1.20	0.88	0.97	1.22	0.86	0.97	1.18	0.87	0.96	1.18	0.89	0.97	1.20	0.88	0.97	1.18
Set2 (SL 1:2)	0.88	0.95	1.20	0.88	0.95	1.20	0.88	0.97	1.20	0.88	0.97	1.19	0.88	0.97	1.19	0.88	0.98	1.19
Set3 (SL 1:3)	0.87	0.96	1.20	0.87	0.96	1.20	0.87	0.98	1.19	0.87	0.98	1.18	0.88	0.98	1.18	0.87	0.96	1.20
Set4 (SL 2:1)	0.89	0.97	1.22	0.86	0.97	1.22	0.88	0.97	1.23	0.89	0.97	1.22	0.89	0.98	1.22	0.89	0.97	1.22
Set5 (SL 3:1)	0.90	0.98	1.20	0.88	0.98	1.23	0.88	0.98	1.22	0.88	0.98	1.20	0.88	0.98	1.20	0.89	0.98	1.20
Average	0.88	0.96	1.20	0.87	0.97	1.21	0.87	0.97	1.20	0.88	0.97	1.19	0.88	0.98	1.20	0.88	0.97	1.20

Not significant

Table 27.0 : The interaction effects of temperature, sources of milk, fat, SNF and starter culture on lactic acid content (%) of yoghurt

Temperature x Sources of milk x Fat x SNF — M₁ (Cow milk)

Starter culture	T₁ (39°C) F₁ (4%) S1 (10%)	S2 (11%)	S3 (12%)	F₂ (5%) S1 (10%)	S2 (11%)	S3 (12%)	F₃ (6%) S1 (10%)	S2 (11%)	S3 (12%)	T₂ (42°C) F₁ (4%) S1 (10%)	S2 (11%)	S3 (12%)	F₂ (5%) S1 (10%)	S2 (11%)	S3 (12%)	F₃ (6%) S1 (10%)	S2 (11%)	S3 (12%)
Set1 (SL 1:1)	0.85	0.87	0.90	0.85	0.87	0.90	0.85	0.87	0.90	0.87	0.88	0.94	0.88	0.88	0.94	0.87	0.88	0.94
Set2 (SL 1:2)	0.86	0.88	0.91	0.86	0.88	0.91	0.86	0.88	0.91	0.88	0.89	0.95	0.89	0.89	0.96	0.88	0.89	0.96
Set3 (SL 1:3)	0.86	0.90	0.92	0.87	0.90	0.92	0.86	0.90	0.92	0.89	0.95	0.97	0.95	0.95	0.97	0.89	0.95	0.97
Set4 (SL 2:1)	0.99	1.07	1.10	0.99	1.08	1.10	0.99	1.08	1.10	1.03	1.11	1.13	1.02	1.12	1.13	1.03	1.12	1.13
Set5 (SL 3:1)	1.00	1.06	1.11	1.00	1.10	1.12	1.10	1.10	1.12	1.16	1.13	1.14	1.12	1.13	1.15	1.13	1.14	1.16
Average	0.91	0.96	0.99	0.91	0.97	0.99	0.91	0.97	0.99	0.96	0.99	1.02	0.96	0.99	1.03	0.96	1.00	1.03

Temperature x Sources of milk x Fat x SNF — M₂ (Buffalo milk)

Starter culture	T₁ (39°C) F₁ (4%) S1 (10%)	S2 (11%)	S3 (12%)	F₂ (5%) S1 (10%)	S2 (11%)	S3 (12%)	F₃ (6%) S1 (10%)	S2 (11%)	S3 (12%)	T₂ (42°C) F₁ (4%) S1 (10%)	S2 (11%)	S3 (12%)	F₂ (5%) S1 (10%)	S2 (11%)	S3 (12%)	F₃ (6%) S1 (10%)	S2 (11%)	S3 (12%)
Set1 (SL 1:1)	0.85	0.88	0.91	0.86	0.88	0.96	0.86	0.88	0.91	0.87	0.88	0.95	2.88	0.89	0.95	0.88	0.89	0.96
Set2 (SL 1:2)	0.86	0.88	0.92	0.86	0.88	0.92	0.87	0.88	0.92	0.88	0.90	0.95	0.88	0.89	0.96	0.88	0.89	0.96
Set3 (SL 1:3)	0.87	0.91	0.94	0.87	0.91	0.94	0.87	0.92	0.64	0.89	0.96	0.98	0.89	0.96	0.98	0.89	0.96	0.99
Set4 (SL 2:1)	0.99	1.08	1.10	1.00	1.06	1.10	1.00	1.06	1.11	1.04	1.13	1.12	1.03	1.13	1.13	1.04	1.13	1.14
Set5 (SL 3:1)	1.00	1.10	1.14	1.00	1.10	1.14	1.02	1.11	1.14	1.11	1.15	1.15	1.12	1.15	1.16	1.12	1.16	1.17
Average	0.91	0.97	1.00	0.92	0.97	1.00	0.92	0.97	1.00	0.96	1.00	1.03	0.96	1.00	1.04	0.96	1.01	1.04

Not significant

Table 27.1 : The interaction effect of temperature, sources of milk, fat, SNF and starter culture on pH of yoghurt

Temperature x Sources of milk x Fat x SNF — M₁ (Cow milk)

| Starter culture | T₁ (39°C) | | | | | | | | | T₂ (42°C) | | | | | | | | |
| | F₁ (4%) | | | F₂ (5%) | | | F₃ (6%) | | | F₁ (4%) | | | F₂ (5%) | | | F₃ (6%) | | |
	S1 (10%)	S2 (11%)	S3 (12%)	S1 (10%)	S2 (11%)	S3 (12%)	S1 (10%)	S2 (11%)	S3 (12%)	S1 (10%)	S2 (11%)	S3 (12%)	S1 (10%)	S2 (11%)	S3 (12%)	S1 (10%)	S2 (11%)	S3 (12%)
Set1 (SL 1:1)	4.85	4.64	4.60	4.78	4.63	4.58	4.77	4.70	4.59	4.66	4.61	4.56	4.60	4.61	4.56	4.62	4.61	4.56
Set2 (SL 1:2)	4.80	4.62	4.58	4.70	4.60	4.58	4.68	4.61	4.58	4.63	4.58	4.55	4.61	4.59	4.55	4.61	4.59	4.55
Set3 (SL 1:3)	4.67	4.60	4.57	4.68	4.70	4.57	4.66	4.59	4.57	4.60	4.56	4.54	4.60	4.55	4.54	4.60	4.55	4.54
Set4 (SL 2:1)	4.54	4.45	4.50	4.54	4.46	4.44	4.54	4.45	4.44	4.51	4.52	4.42	4.52	4.44	4.43	4.52	4.44	4.42
Set5 (SL 3:1)	4.52	4.44	4.44	4.53	4.44	4.43	4.53	4.43	4.43	4.38	4.42	4.41	4.44	4.43	4.36	4.43	4.41	4.38
Average	4.68	4.55	4.54	4.65	4.57	4.52	4.64	4.56	4.52	4.56	4.54	4.50	4.56	4.52	4.49	4.56	4.52	4.49

Temperature x Sources of milk x Fat x SNF — M₂ (Buffalo milk)

| Starter culture | T₁ (39°C) | | | | | | | | | T₂ (42°C) | | | | | | | | |
| | F₁ (4%) | | | F₂ (5%) | | | F₃ (6%) | | | F₁ (4%) | | | F₂ (5%) | | | F₃ (6%) | | |
	S1 (10%)	S2 (11%)	S3 (12%)	S1 (10%)	S2 (11%)	S3 (12%)	S1 (10%)	S2 (11%)	S3 (12%)	S1 (10%)	S2 (11%)	S3 (12%)	S1 (10%)	S2 (11%)	S3 (12%)	S1 (10%)	S2 (11%)	S3 (12%)
Set1 (SL 1:1)	4.80	4.62	4.58	4.78	4.61	4.58	4.76	4.60	4.58	4.62	4.61	4.56	4.62	4.61	4.56	4.61	4.60	4.56
Set2 (SL 1:2)	4.70	4.60	4.57	4.69	4.60	4.57	4.68	4.60	4.57	4.61	4.58	4.56	4.60	4.59	4.55	4.60	4.59	4.55
Set3 (SL 1:3)	4.66	4.59	4.57	4.65	4.58	4.56	4.65	4.57	4.56	4.60	4.55	4.54	4.60	4.55	4.54	4.60	4.55	4.54
Set4 (SL 2:1)	4.54	4.46	4.50	4.54	4.45	4.50	4.53	4.44	4.44	4.51	4.43	4.44	4.51	4.43	4.43	4.51	4.42	4.43
Set5 (SL 3:1)	4.52	4.44	4.43	4.53	4.44	4.42	4.53	4.43	4.42	4.43	4.41	4.40	4.44	4.41	4.38	4.43	4.40	4.36
Average	4.64	4.54	4.53	4.64	4.54	4.53	4.63	4.53	4.51	4.55	4.52	4.50	4.55	4.52	4.49	4.55	4.51	4.49

Not significant

Phase-II

In order to test the hypothesis if the feeding of yoghurt has any growth stimulating and hypocholesteric effects in human beings, an animal experimentation was conducted in the second section of thesis. To meet out objectives, thirty albino rats were obtained at the age of 4 weeks. The animals were maintained in the laboratory in a suitable room, having proper facilities. The rats were fed a diet prepared in our laboratory having a mixture of ground wheat, soyabean and oat. The diet on an average contained 15% proteins. The rats were kept on this diet for at least 7-8 days for proper adaptation. After the adaptation, period, rats were randomly divided into five groups of six each.

Rats were housed in five metal cages, having one group in each. The metallic cages were kept in the laboratory having a temperature of $26^{0}C$ and approximate humidity of 50 to 60 percent and maintained in a cycle of 12 hr. light and 12 hr. dark. The rats in group I, received only the normal diet as described in previous paragraphs and was designated as control group. Group2 rats, in addition to the diet, also received 10% of milk. The rats in groups, 3,4 and 5 were given original ration plus 10, 20 and 30% of yoghurt respectively. The contents of milk or yoghurt were thoroughly mixed in the ration in order to have uniform intake. Enough water was provided to all the groups of rats.

The rats were fed their assigned diets ad libitum for 32 days. Food intake was recorded at an interval of 4 days. Body weights of these rats were recorded individually at the beginning and end of the study.

4.3 Feed intake

The effects of dietary milk and yoghurt in various proportions on food intake in rats are shown in table-27.2. The average intake of rats irrespective of treatments at the start of the experiment was 35 gm/rat, that reached to the

Table 27.2 :   Effect of feeding yoghurt on feed intake in rats

Group/Treatments	4 days	8 days	12 days	16 days	20 days	24 days	28 days	32 days	Mean
Group A (Control	28.50	30.00	32.50	28.33	37.50	37.50	39.16	40.83	34.29
Group B (Control + 10% milk)	30.00	36.25	38.33	37.50	41.66	36.66	40.00	42.50	37.86
Group C (Control + 10% yoghurt)	32.50	38.00	40.00	38.33	49.16	42.50	45.00	46.66	41.52
Group D (Control + 20% yoghurt)	36.50	40.0	45.00	42.50	50.83	44.16	46.33	45.00	43.85
Group E (Control + 30% yoghurt)	47.50	51.50	55.33	48.16	55.83	54.16	50.00	50.33	51.66
Mean	35.00	39.25	42.33	38.96	46.99	42.99	44.09	45.06	

CD for treatment at 5% = 2.46, at 1% = 3.32

Table 27.3 :   Effect of feeding yoghurt on body weight in rats

Group/Treatments	0 days	4 days	8 days	12 days	16 days	20 days	24 days	28 days	32 days
Group A (Control	45.00	54.17	65.83	75.00	79.17	84.17	90.00	93.00	98.0
Group B (Control + 10% milk)	37.50	45.83	59.17	65.50	70.67	78.33	83.67	88.33	95.50
Group C (Control + 10% yoghurt)	38.33	48.33	60.83	66.33	72.50	81.67	87.50	96.17	106.00
Group D (Control + 20% yoghurt)	41.67	56.67	67.50	75.83	82.50	93.33	98.67	103.67	107.17
Group E (Control + 30% yoghurt)	36.67	47.50	60.83	70.83	79.17	91.67	98.67	103.50	110.00

Not significant

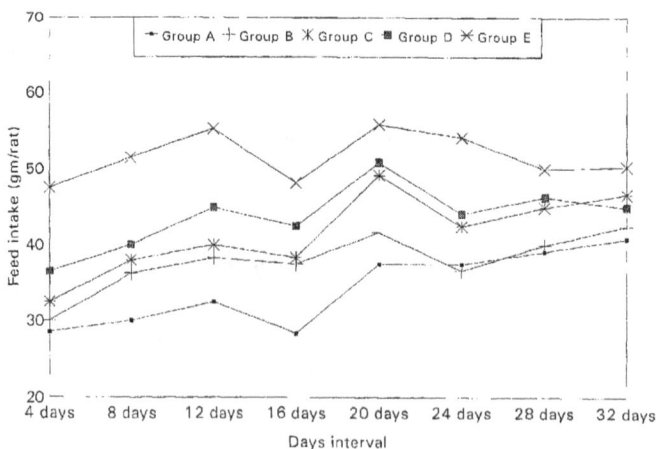

Fig. 4.1: Effect of feeding yoghurt on feed intake in rats

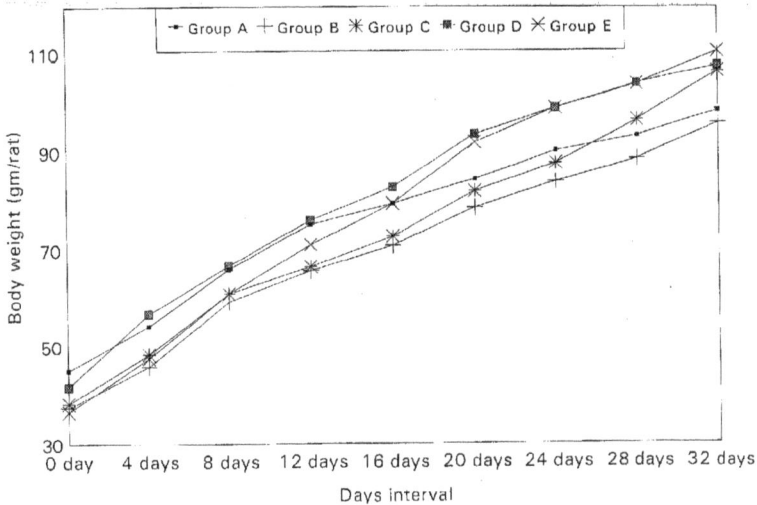

Fig. 4.2: Effect of feeding yoghurt on body weights in rats

extent of 45.06 gm/ratat the end of the experiment. Similarly the average feed efficiency ratio for the combined rats was calculated to be 5.36. Supplementation of either milk or yoghurt resulted in higher feed intake. The results were found to be significant (P < 0.01). As the proportions of yoghurt increased in the diet the food intake also increased. This trend of increasing food intake in yoghurt diets was recorded right from the 4th day of experiment. At four day period the controlled groups on an average ate only 28.50 gm/rat as compared to 30 gms in milk diet. This feed intake reached to 32.50, 36.50 and 47.50 gm in diets supplemented with 10, 20 and 30% of yoghurt. The statistical analysis could not depict much variations in the groups of rats kept on controlled diet and on diet supplemented with 10% milk.

The graphic representations of feed intake data (Fig.-4.1) in all the five groups of rats have clearly depicted the trend of feed intakes. A general trend of feed intakes in all the groups of rats showed that the feed intakes had almost a linear trend up to 20 days period, although the variations within the groups were more apparent. From 20 days to 32 days period the trend of increase in feed intake became almost constant. More surprisingly the feed intakes for group 4, 5 declined from 20 days to 32 days period. The intake in rest of the three groups remained almost constant. The feed intake in rats receiving 30% yoghurt in their diet started with higher intake at 4 days period (47.5 gms), and remained higher (50.33 gm) at 32 at period, in comparison to rats in rest of the groups.

4.4 Weight gain

The effects of diet supplementation with milk and various levels of yoghurt on changes in body weights of rats, along with weight gain, and feed efficiency ratio have been given in table 27.3 and 27.4. The pattern of changes in weight of these rats from 0 days period have been illustrated in graph (Fig.-4.2).

Table 27.4 : Effect of feeding yoghurt on body weight gain and feed efficiency of rats

Group/Treatments	Body weight gain (gm)	Feed efficiency (quantity of feed/gm gain in weight)
Group A (Control)	53.00	5.76
Group B (Control + 10% milk)	58.00	5.53
Group C (Control + 10% yoghurt)	67.67	5.16
Group D (Control + 20% yoghurt)	65.50	5.19
Group E (Control + 30% yoghurt)	73.33	5.19

CD for weight gain at 5% = 1.33, at 1% = N.S.

Feed efficiency-non significant

Table 27.5 : Effect of feeding yoghurt on some blood profiles in rats (Serum cholesterol, sugar, triglyceride and phospholipids)

As can be seen from the table (Table 27.4) the rats that were

Group/Treatments	Blood Profiles			
	Cholesterol (mg/100 ml)	Sugar (mg/100 ml)	Triglyceride (mg/dl)	Phospholipids (mg/100 ml)
Group A (Control)	61.59	48.54	86.00	6.82
Group B (Control + 10% milk)	65.50	81.06	89.00	8.68
Group C (Control + 10% yoghurt)	53.10	97.57	88.00	7.75
Group D (Control + 20% yoghurt)	51.97	87.37	85.00	8.68
Group E (Control + 30% yoghurt)	50.80	86.30	83.00	8.06
SD	± 5.85	±16.69	±2.14	± 0.69
CD at 5%	0.71	2.09	2.34	0.24
CD at 1%	1.02	3.05	3.41	0.35

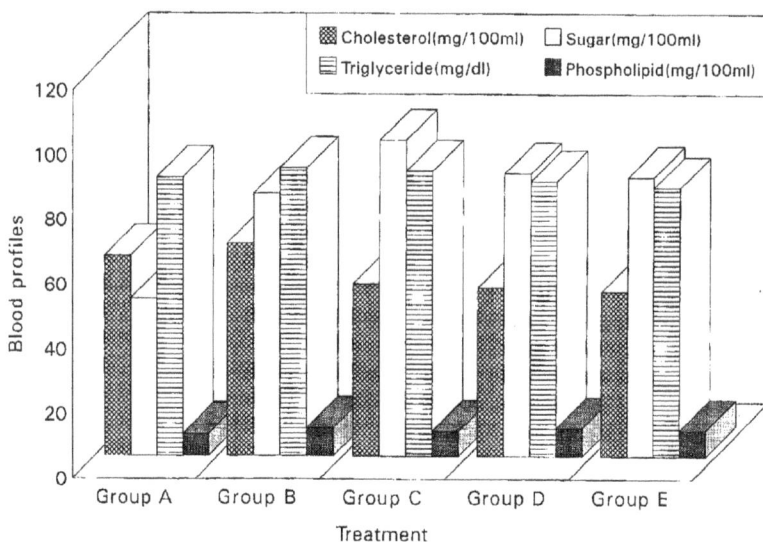

Fig. 4.3: Effect of feeding yoghurt on some blood profile in rats

fed yoghurt along with basal diet had higher average weight gain than did the control group. Differences in weight gains among all the five groups were highly significant (P < 0.01). The maximum weight gain of 73.33 gms in 32 days period was observed in rats receiving 30% of yoghurt followed by those receiving 10% (67.67 gms) and 20% (65.50 gms) yoghurt in their diets. The differences in weight gain in rats receiving diet either with 10 or 20% yoghurt did not prove to be significant. Similarly the weight gain of 53 gms in rats with basal ration and those having 10% milk supplementation (58.00 gms) were not found to be at variance.

4.5 Feed efficiency

When feed intake and gain in weigh were assessed in terms of feed efficiency (Table 27.4), the diets supplemented with 20 or 30% yoghurt resulted in maximum feed efficiency of 5.19, in comparison to either control group (5.76), or the one supplemented with milk (5.53). The later two groups did not differ significantly. Similarly in terms of feed efficiency no differences were noticed between diets with different properties of yoghurt (20% and 30%). Thus this study has indicated the presence of growth stimulant in yoghurt.

The graphic representation of the data clearly depicted the growth pattern of rats from all the five groups. No doubts the rats were divided randomly amongst the five groups, the rats on an average weight only 36 gms in the group receiving 30% yoghurt alongwith basal diet comparatively lesser than the rats in rest of the groups. But on account of faster growth rate in this groups, the rats in this group surpassed rest of the rats in respect to their body weight. This clearly indicated that the yoghurt might have some stimulating factor for growth.

The present study has clearly indicated that the rats receiving yoghurt supplemented diets had a higher feed intake than the rats kept on either in control basal diet or the one supplemented with 10% milk. No doubt the voluntary food intake (VFI) is a function of the hypothalamic control of feed intake, the kind of food may also affect the VFI to a large, as has been the case in present study.

It seems the VFI in rats having diets supplemented with different proportions of yoghurt was because of the quality of food, as the rats in all the groups were from the same origin and of the same age and were also given the diet ad libitum. Since five groups of diets were not made iso-caloric, this could be one of the reasons for higher intake in rats with yoghurt diets.

Higher feed intake in a rats as observed in our study has also been substantiated with the study of Hitchins *et al.* (1983), who in their study have reported that stimulation of weaning rat growth by yoghurt and related fermented milk is associated with increased feed consumption and increased feed efficiency. It is not only that the superiority of yoghurt has been established over controlled diet without yoghurt, but the yoghurt has been proved to be better in terms of growth rate and feed efficiency than other fermented products (Hargrove and Alford, 1978). These authors when fed yoghurt and three other types of acidophilus milk, lactic butter milk, Bulgarian butter milk and directly acidified milk to rats in 6 different trials, observed that yoghurt gave greater weight gains than uninoculated control and other fermented milks. According to Mc Donough *et al.* (1982), the weight gains of rats on yoghurt were 24.3% higher than for milk.

4.6 Blood profile

The effects of feeding yoghurt along with basal ration on serum lipids and glucose levels are shown in table 27.5. Simultaneously the variations in concentrations of various lipids fractions and glucose level as affected by feeding various amounts of yoghurt have been presented through the bar diagram (Fig.-4.3).

The total serum cholesterol levels in rats on basal diet and in these supplemented with 30% yoghurt were 61.59 and 50.80 per cent respectively. The differences in reduction of cholesterol level was to the extent of 17.52 per cent when the diet was supplement with 30% yoghurt (diet E). The extent of reduction in cholesterol declined to 15.62% when yoghurt supplementation was 20%, which further declined to 13.78% when the yoghurt was mixed to the extent of 10%. The reduction in cholesterol levels in blood of the rats maintained on yoghurt diets over the control groups were statistically significant (P < 0.01). As the yoghurt increased in the diet the cholesterol level got reduced but the variations in the cholesterol level of blood from rats maintained in diets C, D and E were not significant. Surprisingly. Addition of whole milk in the diet (group B) to the extent of 10% caused a significant increase in cholesterol level from 61.59 to 65.50% resulting an increase of 6.35%.

High concentration of total cholesterol is highly associated with an increased risk of coronary heart disease. Reduction in total cholesterol in hypercholesterolemic men reduces the incidence of cardiovascular disease. Modification of diets, such as supplementation of diet with fermented dairy products like yoghurt or lactic acid bacteria-containing dairy products is one way that the serum cholesterol may be reduced.

This has clearly been demonstrated through our study with experimental rats. The bacteria in yoghurt or any other lactic acid producing bacteria may alter serum cholesterol level by two proposed mechanisms (Usma & Hosono, 2000). Firstly by directly binding dietary cholesterol into the small intestine before the cholesterol can be absorbed into the body and secondly by deconjugating bile acid to produce free bile acid. The present study with rats are in agreement with work reported earlier (Danielson *et al.*, 1989 and Navder *et al.*, 1990). A lot of variations have been reported by these authors. The main cause of variations are the groups of microorganisms. Contrary to may studies as reported above including ours authors like Grunewald & Mitchel (1983) have reported that acidophilus milk had no effect on serum cholesterol in mice.

Supplementation of 10% milk in the diet could not cause any reduction in the serum cholesterol level is rats, rather it caused about 6.35% increase in cholesterol level. Very conflicting reports regarding feeding of milk on blood parameters in man and experimental animals are available. According to Usam & Hosono (2000) dietary milk had no effects on total cholesterol & LDL cholesterol. Similar observation have also been reported by Grunewald (1982) and Mann (1978). Contrary to these findings Keim *et al.* (1981) reported reduction in HDL cholesterol in human receiving diets either with yoghurt or milk. Since in our study we did not bifurcate LDL & HDL cholesterol, no comparison can be make. But in our study with rats milk to the extent of 10% of diet in rats caused an increase in total cholesterol from 61.59% to 65.50%.

Supplementation of diets with either milk or yoghurt resulted in small but not significant changes in serum triglyceride levels in rat's serum. No consistent changes were seen between diets with or without milk or yoghurt. The rats on basal diet had on an average of 86.0% triglycerides that declined to 83.00% in diet with 30% yoghurt that was significant. The triglyceride levels with diets having 10 or 20% yoghurt were 88.00 & 85.0% respectively. These values were very irregular and also insignificant. Feeding milk also could not change the triglyceride levels in rats in this experiment. A small but non-significant decline in triglyceride was also observed by Aklin *et al.* (1997), in mice having acidophilus diet.

Similar results were also observed by Danidson *et al.* (1970) in mature boars fed acidophilus yoghurt and by Hepner *et al.* (1979) in human fed yoghurt. However, Jones *et al.* (1985) have found that yoghurt had lowered triglyceride concentrations of piglets. Moussa *et al.* (1995) found that both yoghurt and acidophilus yoghurt had the same effects on triglyceride concentration of rats.

The data related to changes in serum phospholipids in rats kept on various diets supplemented with milk and yoghurt are presented in table 27.5. Histogram showing concentration of phospholipids and other lipid constituents are given in Fig. – 4.3. In rats having basal diet without milk or yoghurt supplementation, the level of phospholipids was 6.82 mg/100 ml. This value was elevated to the extent of 8.68 mg/100 ml in B and D groups of rats that were fed 10% milk and 20% yoghurt in addition to basal diets. These variations were found to be statistically significant ($P < 0.01$). The level of yoghurt feeding did not seem to have any specific effects on serum phospholipids, as the increase was very much erratic, as can be observed from the table 27.5.

Increased feed intake might have resulted in increase of serum phospholipids levels in experimental rats.

The concentration of blood glucose levels in five groups of rats kept on five different diets are presented in table 27.5 & their diagrammatic presentations have been depicted in the histogram (Fig. 4.2). The blood glucose level; in control group was only 48.54 mg/100 ml that rose to 81.06 mg/100 ml, when the diet was supplemented with 10% milk. Similarly the addition of 10% yoghurt in diet allowed the blood glucose level to rose to the extent of 97.57 mg/100 ml., that declined slowly as the levels of yoghurt was increased in the diet. This can clearly be observed through the histograms. The variations in blood-glucose levels were found to be statistically significant ($P < 0.01$).

Since the diets in question were not made iso-caloric : Certainly the diets with higher intake and with high calories/gm might have resulted in higher concentration of blood-glucose levels.

9 Summary and Conclusion

Yoghurt is a western fermented milk product, originated in western Europe. It is similar to dahi prepared in our country. Now a days yoghurt is gaining more popularity in our country, but the appropriate scientific information about manufacture of yoghurt and its nutritional impact are still lacking. Therefore, it was thought to prepare yoghurt from different levels of fat, SNF & bacteria in cow and buffalo milk inoculated at two levels of temperature. The nutritional performance of best quality yoghurt was judged by a feeding experiment on rats.

The entire experiments were carried out in two phases (kumar,2002) - In phase-I, cow and buffalo milk were standardized with three levels of fat viz., 4% (F1). 5% (F2), & 6% (F3) and SNF viz., 10% (S1), 11% (S2) & 12% (S3). All the standardized milk samples were treated with S. thermophilus (S) and L.bulgaricus (L) in five levels of starter culture viz., Set$_1$ (SL 1 : 1), Set$_2$ (SL 1 : 2), Set$_3$ (SL 1: 3), Set$_4$ (SL 2 : 1) & Set$_5$ (SL 3 : 1) and incubated at 39°C (T1) and 42°C (T2), separately for the preparation of yoghurt. The yoghurt samples were judged by a panel of five judges to findout the effects of above factors on physical attributes (flavour, body & texture, acidity, score and colour & appearance), of yoghurt. The yoghurt samples were also chemically examined.

In phase-II, 30 albino rats were selected at the age of one moth, and devided randomly equally into five groups viz. , group A (basal diet), group B (basal diet + 10% milk), group C (basal diet + 10% yoghurt), group D (basal diet + 20 % yoghurt) and group E (basal diet + 30% yoghurt). After 32 days of feeding trial, blood samples of individual rat were collected for the analysis of serum cholesterol, serum triglyceride, serum glucose and serum phospholipids.

The results obtained in the present study are summarized here under :

Phase- I

A - Physical Attributes

The flavour, body & texture, acidity and colour and appearance of cow milk yoghurt were 36.71, 24.80, 11.17 and 3.56 respectively. The respective value for buffalo milk yoghurt were 36.27, 25.16, 11.25 and 3.83 respectively. The flavour score (36.71) of cow milk yoghurt was significantly ($P < 0.01$) higher than the flavour score (36.27) of buffalo milk yoghurt. Whereas the body & texture, acidity and colour & appearance score of buffalo milk yoghurt was significantly ($P < 0.01$ higher than the cow milk yoghurt. The overall score (81.51) of buffalo milk yoghurt was higher than the overall score (81.24) of cow milk yoghurt.

The flavour score of yoghurt increased significantly ($P < 0.01$) from 33.72 to 39.26 when temperature was increased from 39°C to 42°C. Similarly, body & texture increased from 24.77 to 25.20, acidity from 11.13 to 11.29 and colour & appearance from 3.67 to 3.72 when temperature was increased from 39°C to 42°C. The overall acceptablity score was higher for yoghurt prepared at higher temperature than overall acceptability score (78.29) of yoghurt prepared at lower temperature.

The flavour score was significantly ($P < 0.01$), higher in yoghurt from cow milk as compared to the value observed in buffalo milk yoghurt at both incubation temperature. The best flavour was observed in cow milk yoghurt prepared at 42°C.

The flavour and body & texture scores of yoghurt samples prepared at both the temperatures increased ($P < 0.01$) with increasing concentration of fat in the milk. The maximum flavour (40.73) and body & texture score (25.51) were recorded in the sample prepared at 42°C in association with 6% fat in milk.

The flavour, body & texture quality of yoghurt significantly (P < 0.01) improved as the SNF content increased in the milk, irrespective of starter culture used. The maximum flavour and body & texture score was observed when the sample was prepared with the 12% SNF and 6% fat.

The flavour score increased significantly (P < 0.01) as the concentration of lactobacilli increased in the milk, but the values abruptly declined (P < 0.01) even from the normal (SL 1 : 1) when the levels of streptococci increased in the culture.

The respective average scores of flavour, body & texture, acidity and colour & appearance were 34.65, 24.71, 11.09 and 3.44 in the samples prepared with 4.0% fat; 36.51, 25.20, 11.35 and 3.94 in the samples prepared from milk containing 6.0% fat.

Flavour and textural quality of yoghurt improved significantly (P < 0.01) as the concentration of lactobacilli and fat increased in the milk whereas, the values dropped significantly (P < 0.01) as the proportions of streptococci increased in the culture.

The average score of flavour, body & texture, acidity and colour & appearance were 35.88, 23.28, 11.05 and 3.56 in yoghurt prepared from milk containing 10% SNF; 36.37, 24.51, 11.21 and 3.68 in the sample prepared with 11.0% SNF in milk and 37.19, 27.17, 11.38 and 3.85 in the samples prepared with 12.0% SNF in milk. All the physical attributes increased significantly (P < 0.01) as the concentration of SNF increases in the milk. Yoghurt prepared from milk containing 12.0% SNF proved to be the best in respect of flavour, body & texture, acidity and colour & appearance of yoghurt.

All the physical attributes, except colour & appearance of yoghurt, significantly (P < 0.01) increased as the levels of lactobacilli increased in the milk, but the same was not true when the proportions of S. thermophilus enhanced in the culture. The values of these physical attributes decreased significantly (P < 0.01) as the levels of streptococci increased in the culture and vice-versa. With increasing the levels of loctobacilli in M_1 and M_2, the flavour score of yughurt also increased significantly (P < 0.01). This trend reversed when the levels of streptococci was enhanced in the culture.

The flavour & texture quality of yoghurt prepared from cow and buffalo milk at 39°C and 42°C improved significantly (P < 0.01) as the concentration of SNF increased in the milk. The flavour score of yoghurt enhanced (P < 0.01) with increasing the concentration of lactobacilli, irrespective of temperature and type of milk used. The combined effects of temperature, sources of milk and starter culture on body & texture, colour & appearance and acidity were not significant.

The flavour, body & texture, colour & appearance and acidity of yoghurt apparently increased with increasing levels of temperature, fat and SNF. The flavour score of yoghurt increased significantly (P < 0.01) as fat content and lactobacilli increased in the milk, irrespective of culture and temperature used. But, the flavour quality of yoghurt reduced significantly (P < 0.01) as the proportions of streptococci increased in the culture.

The body & texture quality of yoghurt, prepared from cow and buffalo milk increased with increasing levels of SNF in milk, irrespective of the starter culture used.

The flavour score of cow and buffalo milk yoghurt prepared at both temperature increased significantly (P < 0.01) with increase in the concentration of fat in milk, irrespective of starter culture used. The interaction effect of temperature, sources of milk, fat and starter culture on body & texture, acidity and colour & appearance of yoghurt were statistically not significant.

On the basis of physico-chemical observations recorded from the yoghurt samples in the present study, it can be said that the best quality of yoghurt can be prepared with buffalo milk having overall score of 81.24. The quality of yoghurt prepared from the milk having 6% fat and 12% SNF proved to be the best. The starter culture having a ratio of 1: 3 (S & L) and incubation of 42°C were recorded to be optimum for better quality yoghurt.

B. Chemical attributes

The sources of milk and temperature did not effect the fat, protein and ash content of yoghurt. The variations were observed only in lactose, acidity and pH of yoghurt. The lactose (5.32%) and acidity (0.98%) value in buffalo milk yoghurt were significantly (< 0.01) higher than the values observed in cow milk (5.19% and 0.97%), whereas the buffalo milk yoghurt was significantly ($P < 0.01$) lower in respect of pH value (4.54) than the value observed in cow milk (4.55) yoghurt. The lactose content (5.19%) and pH values (4.52) in yoghurt prepared at higher temperature were significantly ($P < 0.01$) lower than the lactose (5.32%) and pH value (4.57) of yoghurt made at lower temperature.

The interaction effects of T x M, and T x F on fat, protein, lactose, ash, acidity and pH of yoghurt were not significant. The acidity of yoghurt significantly ($P < 0.01$) increased as the concentration of SNF increased in the milk during preparation of yoghurt at both the temperature levels, whereas the pH value of yoghurt decreased significantly as SNF concentration in milk increased, irrespective of the temperature. The interaction effect of temperature and SNF on fat, protein, lactose and ash content of yoghurt were statistically not significant.

The average fat content in yoghurt increased from 4.02% to 6.02% ($P < 0.01$) when the levels of fat increased from 4% to 6% in the milk, but the other chemical constituents (protein, lactose, ash and acidity of yoghurt) did not differ significantly with increase or decrease in fat contents of milk. The values for fat, protein, lactose, ash, lactic acid and pH were 4.02%, 4.71%, 5.25%, 1.02%, 0.98% and 4.55% respectively in the yoghurt prepared with 4.0% fat; 5.02%, 4.72%, 5.28%, 1.02%, 0.98% and 4.55 in sample prepared with 5.0% fat and 6.02%, 4.72%, 5.22%, 1.02%, 0.98% and 4.54% in the sample prepared from milk containing 6% fat. The pH value of yoghurt significantly ($P < 0.05$) decreased from 4.55 to 4.54 when fat content in milk increased from 5.0 to 6.0 per cent.

The protein content of yoghurt increased from 4.29% to 5.19% as the concentration of SNF increased from 10% to 12% in the milk. Similarly, the lactose, ash and acidity content of yoghurt also increased from 4.81% to 5.70%, 0.88% to 1.20% and 0.94% to 1.01%, respectively when concentration of SNF increased from 10% to 12% in milk. The pH value of yoghurt was inversely proportion to the SNF content in milk.

Least variations were observed in fat, protein and ash contents of yoghurt prepared from different levels of bacterial inoculation in the milk. The average lactose content in yoghurt were 5.19, 5.38, 5.56, 5.13 and 5.01 per cent when the samples were inoculated with culture group Set_1, Set_2, Set_3. Set_4 and Set_5 respectively. These samples contained 0.89, 0.90, 0.92, 1.08 and 1.11 percent acidity whereas, pH values of yoghurt were recorded as 4.63, 4.61, 4.59, 4.47 and 4.44 in culture group Set1, Set2, Set3, Set4 and Set5 respectively. The average lactic acid content of yoghurt increased significantly ($P < 0.01$) as the proportions of either lactobacilli or streptococci increased in the milk, Where as the pH values reduced significantly as the concentrations of these two bacteria increased in the culture.

Phase - II

The average feed intake in rats/head/day were 8.57, 9.46, 10.38, 10.96 and 12.92 gm in groups A, B, C, D & E respectively. Enhancing the amount of milk and yoghurt in the food resulted in higher ($P < 0.01$) dry matter intake in the rats. The maximum weight gain of 73.33 gms at 32nd day of feeding was observed in rats receiving 30% yoghurt followed by those receiving 10% (67.67) and 20% (65.50) yoghurt in their diets. The differences in the weight gains among all the groups were highly significant ($P < 0.01$).

The diets supplemented with 20 or 30% yoghurt resulted in maximum feed efficiency of 5.19, in comparison to either control group (5/76) or on the diet supplemented with milk (5.53). The differences in the feed efficiency ratio within the groups were not significant.

The reduction in total cholesterol levels in blood of rats maintained in yoghurt diets (50.80) over control groups (61.59) were statistically significant (P < 0.01). As the yoghurt increased in the diet cholesterol level got reduced. But the variations in the cholesterol level of blood from rats maintained in diets C, D and E were not significant. Surprisingly, addition of whole milk in the diet (group B) to the extent of 10% caused a significant (P < 0.01) increase in the cholesterol level from 61.59 to 65.50 per cent resulted an increase of 6.35 per cent.

Supplementation of diets with either milk or yoghurt resulted in small but not significant changes in serum triglyceride levels in rat's serum. The rats on basal diet had on an average of 86.0% triglyceride that declined to 83.00% in diet with 30% yoghurt that was significant (P < 0.01). The triglyceride levels with diets having 10 or 20% yoghurt were 88.00 & 85.00%, respectively. These values were very irregular and also insignificant. The levels of yoghurt feeding did not seem to have any specific effects on serum cholesterol level, without much affecting the triglyceride, phospholipic, and sugar levels.

10 References

Abd-Rabo, F.H., Ahmad, N.S.; Abou, D.A.E.; Hassan, F.A.M. (1992). Changes in milk constituents during the manufacture of goat's milk yoghurt. *Egyptian J. Dairy Sci.* **20** (2), 317-328.

Abreu-Penate, M.; Rodriguez, A.; Torres Harnandez, E. and Moran Cuba, J. (1985). Study of the digestibility of proteins in different types of milk. Revista Cubana de Higiency Epidemiologia. **23**(3), 306-310.

Agerholm-Larsen, L.; Raben, A.; Haulrik, N.; Hansen, A.S.; Manders, M. (2000). Effects of 8 week intake of probiotic milk products on risk factors for cardiovascular diseases. *European J. Clin. Nutr.* **54**(4), 288-297.

Ahmed, T.K. (1992).Comparative study on zabadi made from cow and goat milk with or without SMP supplement. *Sudan J. Animal Production.* **5**, 93-102.

Akalin, A.S. Gonc, S. and Duzel, S. (1997). Influence of yoghurt and acidophilus yoghurt on serum cholesterol levels in mice. *J. Dairy Sci.,* **80**(11), 2721-2725.

Akin, M.S. and Konar, A. (1993). A comparative study of physico-chemical and organoleptic qualities of flavoured yoghurt made from cow and goat milk and stored for 15 days. *Turkish J. Agric. and Forestry,* **23**(sup-3), 557-565.

Alm, L. (1982). Effect of fermetation on L(+) and O (-) lactic acid in milk. *J. Dairy Sci.* 65(4), 515-520.

Al-Dahhan, A.H.; Ali, M.M. and Sibo, N.H. (1984). Study of the effect of different kinds of milk on quality of leben. *Iraqi J. Agril. Sci* 'Zanco', **2**(2), 51-59.

Al-Saleh, A.A. and Hammad, Y.A. (1992). Effect of substituting cow milk, fat by different fat and and oils on yoghurt quality. *Annals* of Agricultural Sciences (airo). **37**(2), 467-472.

A.O.A.C. (1970). Association of Official Analytical Chemists, Official Methods of Analysis, Eleventh Edn. Washington, **4**, DC.

Anderson, J.W. and Gilliland, S.E. (1999). Effect of fermented milk (yoghurt) containing lactobacillus acidophilus on serum cholesterol in hypercholesterolemic humans. J. American College of Nutr. **18** (1), 43-50.

Aranjo, W.M.C.; Pires de Freitas, C.; Pires, E.M.P.; and Lima De Oliveria, S. (1988). Using goat milk for making yoghurt. Cited from Food Sci. and Technol. Abstr. **20** (4), 126.

Aslim, B. (1998). Studying on metabolic products and antagonistic effect of combined Lactobacillus bulgaricus and Streptococcus thermophilus cultures. Turk Hiyge in Ve Deneysel Biyologi Dergisi. **55**(1), 17-23.

Astrup, P. (1977). Diet and Heart Disease. Dairy Sci. Abstr. **39**(12), 7397 p. 831.

Abdel-Salam; Ammar, A.S. and Galal,W.K. (2009). Evaluation and properties of formulated low calories functional yoghurt cake. J. of food, Agriculture and Environment. 7(2): 218-221.

Al-Wabel, N.A., Mousa, H.M. ; Orner, O.H. and Abdel-Salam, A.M. (2008). Biological evaluation of aqueous herbal extracts and stirred yoghurt filtrate mixture against alloxan-induced oxidative stress and diabetes in rats. International J. of Pharmacology. **4**(2) : 135-139.

Anjum, M.A.; Tahir R.R.; Rahman, Z.S. and Ahmad, H.S. (2009). Chemical and sensory characteristics of yoghurts prepared by locally isolated and commercially imported starter cultures. Milch-wissenschaft. **64**(4) : 392-395.

Baccignone, Brijid, R.I. and Sarra, C. (1982). Studies on the composition of triglycerides and free fatty acids in yoghurt made using milk from cow, ewes, and goats. Cited from Dairy Sci. Abstr. **45**, 3087.

Blance, B. (1984). IDF Bulletin 179, 33.

Banks, W. and Evans, E.E. (1983). Homogenization in dairy processing. Milk Industry, **85**(1), 104.

Bazzare, T.L.; Wu, S.L. and Yahas, J.A. (1983). Total and HDL - Cholesterol concentrations following yoghurt and clacium supplementation. Nutrition Reports International. **28**(6), 1225-1232.

Becker, F. (1971). Yoghurt and culture production using instant dried skim milk. Ost. Milchw. **76**, 297.

Becker, F. (1971). Yoghurt and culture production using instant dried skim milk. Ost. Milchw. **76**, 297.

Becker, F. (1971). Yoghurt and culture production using instant dried skim milk. Ost. Milchw. **26**. (16), 297-299.

Becker, T. and Puhan, Z. (1989). Effect of different process to increase the milk solids-not-fat content on the rheological properties of yoghurt. Milchuissenschaft. **44** (10), 626-629.

Beena, A. and Prasad, V. (1997). Effect of yoghurt and bifidus yoghurt fortified with skim milk powder, condensed whey and lactose-hydrolysed condensed whey on serum cholesterol and triacylglycerol levels in rats. *J. Dairy Res.* **64**(3), 453-457.

Bozanic, R.; Traxtinik. L. and Maric, O.(2000). Sensory properties and acceptability of yoghurt and aromatized yoghurt from cow and goat milk. Myekarstvo. **50**(3), 199-208.

Brendchang (1987). Structure formation in acid milk gels. Cited from Food Sci. Technol. Abstr. **19**(4), 4P167.

Cardoso Castaneda, F.; Iniguez Rojas, C. and Hombre Morgado, R. De. (1991). Effect of heat treatment on firmness of yoghurt made from buffalo milk. Revista Cubana de Alimentarion Y Nutrition. **5**(2), 114-117.

Chawla, A.K. and Balachandran, R. (1985). Certain technological parameters for commercial production of yoghurt. A Ph.D thesis submitted to Kurukshetra University (Unpublished).

Chawala, A.K. and Balachandran, R. (1993). Studies on yoghurt from buffalo milk effect of different levels of fat on chemical, rheological and sensory characteristics. *Indian J. Dairy Sci.* (5), 220-222.

Chawala, A.K. and Balachandan, R. (1994). Studies on yoghurt buffalo milk; Effect of different solid-not-fat content on chemicla, rheological and sensory characteristics. Indain J. Dairy Sci. **47**(9), 762-765.

Chazinikolau, N. (1985). [Yoghurt] Joghust. German Federal Republic Patent Application. GM 85 14757.

Cho-Al-Ying, F.; Duitschever, C.L. and Buteau, C. (1990). Influence of temp. of incubation of the physico-chemical and sensory quality of yoghurt. Cult. Dairy Prod. J. 25(3), 11-14.

Chopra, C.S.; Mital, B.K. and Singh, S. (1984). Preparation of a yoghurt like product from soybeans. J. Food Sci. and Technol. India. **21**(2), 81-84.

Cottenie, J.(1978). Yoghurt processing in Europe. Cult. Dairy Prod. J., **13**(6).

Danielson, A.D.; Peo, E.R. Jr. Sahani, K.M.; Lewis, A.J.; Whalen, P.J. and Amer, M.A. (1989). Anticholesteremic property of Lactobacillus acidophilus yoghurt fed to mature boars. J. Animal Sci. **67**(4), 966-974.

Daraoui, A. (1984). Progress made in manufacture of fermented milk, use of reconstituted milk. IDF Bullet. **179**, 123-126.

Dolezalek, J. and Vokacova, H. (1981). Effect of technology on the ripening and quality of yoghurt. Vliv technologie na zrani a jakost jogurtoveho mleka. Praumysl potravin. **32**(8), 460-461.

Dordevic, J.; Caric, M. and Anojcic-Birovljev, V. (1973). Manufacture of foamed cultured milks with the addition of fruit. Mljekarstvo. **23**(2), 26-31.

Driessen, F.M.; Kluts, P.B.G. and Kntp, J. (1989). Melkunie Holland (BV) Structure, Fermented milk products having a fat content of 1 to 40% by weight packed in containers and a method for their preparation. European patent application. EP0316031 AZ, 15pp.

EL-Deeb, S.A. and Hassan, H.N. (1987). Effect of partial substitution of milk solids-not-fat with defatted soyflour on the qualities of Zabadi. Alexandria Science Exchange. **8** (1), 87-105.

Farooq, K. and Haquw, Z.U. (1992). Effect of sugar ester on textural properties on non-fat low caloric yoghurt. J. Dairy Sci. **75**(10), 2676-2680.

Galestool, Th. E; Hassing, F. and Verongo, H.A. (1968). Symbiosis in yoghurt stimulation of L. bulgaricus by a factor produced by S. thermophilus. Neth. Milk Dairy J. **22**, 60.

Garg, S.K. (1988). Dahi- a fermented indegenous milk product. Indian Dairyman. **40**(2), 57-60.

Ghosh, J. and Rajorhia, G.S. (1990). Selection of starter culture for production of indigenous Indian fermented milk product (Misti dahi). Lait (Lyon) **70**(2), 147-154.

Goh, J.S.; Chae, Y.S.; Gang, C.G.; Kwon, I.K.; Choi, M.; Lee, S.K.; kim, G.Y. and Ahn, J.K. (1994). Studies on development of ginseng-yoghurt and its helath effect. II. Effect of ginsend-yoghurt on the blood glucose, serum cholesterol and inhibition of cancer in mouse. Korean J. Dairy Sci., **16**(3), 253-261.

Gono, S.; Kilic, S. and Kinik, O. (1988). Properties of yoghurt made with different amount of starter and different incubation temps. Ege, Universites, Ziraat-Fakultesi Dergisi. **25**(1), 1-9.

Grunewald, K.K. (1982). Serum cholesterol levels in rats fed skim milk fermented by Lactobacillus acidophilus. J. Food Sci. **47**, 2078-2079.

Grunewald, K.K. and Mirchell, K. (1983). Serum cholesterol levels in mice fed fermented and unfermented acidophilus milk. J. Food Prot. **46**, 315-318.

Goodburn, K.F. and Halligan, A.C. (1988). Modified atmosphere and active packaging - a technology guide. Publication of British Food manufacturing Research Association, Leatherhead, U.K.

Goldin, S. (1980) J.Dairy Science 63, 1031 cited in Functions of Formented milk by yuji Nakazawa and Akiyoshi Hosono (1992), Elsevier Applied Science, London. 1 Edn, pp14.

Gowder, S.J.T. and Halagowder, D. (2008). Food Flavour cinnamaldehyde-induced biochemical and histological changes in the kidney of male albino wister rat. Environmental Toxicology and Pharma. **26**(1) : 68-74.

Ghadge, P.N.; Prasad, K. and Kadam, P.S. (2008). Effect of fortification on the physico-chemical and sensory properties of buffalo milk yoghurt. Electronic J. of Environmental, Agri and Food chemi. **7**(5) : 2890-2899.

Hui, Y.H. (1993). Dairy Science and Technology Handbook, Vol. 3: Applications Science, Technology, and Engineering, I Edn. New york.

Hui, Y.H. (1993). Dairy Science and Techonology Handbook, Vol. 2: Product Manufacturing, I Edn, New york.

Han, J.H. (2000). Antimicrobial food packaging. Food Technol 54(3) 56-65.

Hamme, D; Wahl, D and Mardi, M: (1980) Le Lait 60, 111. Cited from Nakazava, y. and Hosono, A. (1992). Functions of furmented milk. London

Hargrove, R.E. and Alford, J.A. (1978). Growth rate and feed efficiency of rats fed yoghurt and other fermented milks. J. Dairy Sci. **61**(1), 11-19.

Hargrove R.E. and Alford, J.A. (1978). Growth response in rats fed fermented milks. XX Int. Dairy Cong. Vol. E. 972-973.

Hargrove, R.E. and Alford, J.A. (1980). Growth response of weanling rats to heated, aged, fractionated, and chemically treated yoghurts. J. Dairy Sci., **63**(7), 1065-1072.

Hassan, H.N. and Mistry, V.V. (1991). Production of low fat yoghurt from a high milk protein powder. (Abstr.) J. Dairy Sci. **74** (Supplement I), 96.

Henny, A.A.; Mehriz, A.M., Hassan, M.N.A.and Aziz, A.H. (1995). Effect of different inoculum size and fat percentage on some properties and acceptability of sour acidophilus milk produced from buffalo's milk. Egyptian J. Dairy Sci. **23**(1), 123-134.

Hepner, G.R.; Fried, R.; Leor, S.; Fusetti, L. and Morin, R. (1979). Hypocholesterolemic effect of yoghurt and milk Am. J. Clin. Nutr. **32**, 19.

Higashio, K.; kikuchi, T. and Furuichi, E. (1978). The symbiosis between Lactobacillus bulgaricus and Streptococcus thermophilus in yoghurt cultures. In XX Int. Dairy Cong. Vol E., 515-516.

Hitchins, A.D.; Mc Donough, F.E.; Wong, N.P. and Hargrove, R.E. (1983). Biological and biochemical variables affecting the relative values for growth and feed efficiency of rats fed yoghurt or milk. J. Food Sci. **48**(6), 1836-1840.

Hofi Khorshid, M.A.; Khalil, S.A. and Ismail, A.A. (1994). The use of ultrafiltered whey protein concentrate in the manufacture of zabadi. Egyptian J. Food Sci. **22**(2), 189-200.

Hofi, M.A. (1988). Labneh (concentrated yoghurt) from ultrafiltered milk. Scandinarian Dairy Industry. **2**(1), 50-52.

Hong, B.J. and Goh, J.S. (1979). Effect of temperature and time on pasteurization and fermentation on quality of yoghurt. Korean J. Dairy Sci. **1**(2), 7-12.

Hong, S.M.; Shin, J.H.; Kim, E.R.; Lce, J.I and Yu, J.H. (1995). Effect on the texture and flavours of frozen yoghurt by mixed strain culture. Korean J. Dairy Sci. **17**(3), 206-213.

Humphreys, C.L. and Plunkett (1969). Yoghurt a review of its manufacture. Cited from Dairy Sci. Abstr. **31**, 607.

Iniguez, C.; Cardoso, F. and Hombre, R. DE. (1991). Effect of heat treatment on certain quality aspects of yoghurt manufacture from buffalo skim milk. Alimentaria. **28**(226), 49-51.

IS : 1224 (Part I). (1977). Determination of fat by Gerbar methods in Milk. Indian Standards Institution, Mamak Bhavan, New Delhi.

IS : 1479 (Part I). (1960). Methods of test for dairy industry : Part I Rapid examination of milk. Indian Standard Institution, Manak Bhavan, New Delhi.

IS : 1479 (Part II). (1961). Methods of test for dairy industry : Part II Chemical analysis of milk. Indian Standard Institution, Manak Bhavan, New Delhi.

Ishida, M. and Kubo, H. (1985). Effects of yoghurt, kefir and buttermilk on serum lipids in rats. Scientific Reports of the Miyagi Agricultural College, No. 33, 43-47.

Jaspers, D.A.; Massey, L.K. and Leudecke, L.O (1984). Effect of consuming yoghurts prepared with three culture strains on human serum lipoproteins. J. Food. Sci. **49**(4), 1178-1181.

Jennes, R. and Patton, S. (1959). Principle of Dairy Chemistry, Chapman and Hall Ltd. London, U.K., 230-231.

Jogdand, S.B.; Lembhe, A.F. and Ambadkar, R.K. (1991). A quality dahi (curd) by addition of the additives. Asian J. Dairy Sci. **19**(3), 169-170.

Jogdand, S.B.; Lembhe, A.F.; Ambadkar, R.K. and Chopade, S.S. (1991). Incorporation of additives to improve the quality of dahi. Indian J. Dairy Sci. **44**(7), 459-460.

Jones, G.; Shahani, K.M. and Amer, A.M. (1985). The effect of acidphilus yoghurt on serum cholesterol, triglyceride and lipoprotein levels of weaning pigs. J. Dairy Sci. **68**(Suppl.1), 84(Abstr.).

Kar, T.; Kar, P.; Maiti, P. and Mishra, A.K. (1998). Hypocholesterolemic effect of acidophilus yoghurt. Environment-and- Ecology. **16**(1), 117-122.

Kaup, S. M. (1988). Bioavailability of calcium in yoghurt and its relationship to the hypocholesterolemic properties of yoghurt. Dissertation-Abstracts-International, B. **48**(7), 1859.

Kehagias, C.; Komiotis, A.; Konlouris, S. and Korain, H. (1987). Physico-chemical properties of set type yoghurt made from cow's, ewe's and goat's milk. Cited from Food Sci. Technol. Abstr. **19**(7), 7P189.

Kehagias, C.; Zervoudaki, A. and Parlama, C. (1989). Influene of composition and additives on properties of set-type yoghurt from goat milk. Small Ruminant Res. **2**(1), 35 - 45.

Kehagias, H.H.; Konidare, P.E.; Laskarts, H.I. and Kazazes, I.S. (1987). Fermentation of cow's, goat's and ewe's milk by thermophilic acid producing cultures. Episteme Kai Tehnologia Galaktos. **4**(1), 43-59.

Keim, N.L. Marlett, J.A. and Amundsopn, C.H. (1981). The cholesterolemic effect of skim milk in young men consuming controlled diets. Nutr. Res. **1**, 429-442.

Khanna, A. and Jasjit Singh, A. (1979). Comparison of yoghurt starter in cow's and buffalo milk. J. Dairy Res. **46**(4), 681-686.

Kheadr, E.E.; Abd-El-Rahman, A.M. and El-Soukkary, F.A.H. (2000). Impact of yoghurt and probiotic strains on serum cholesterol and lipoportein profiles in rats. Alexandria, J. Agril Res. **45**(3), 81-100.

Kilic, S. (1986). Characteristics of yoghurt made with lipid, frozen and freeze-dried cultures containint L. bulgaricus and S. thermophilus bacteria of different origins and properties and in different proportions. Ege Universitesi Zirocet Fakultesi Dergisi **23**(2), 93-104.

King, E.J. and Woofen, W.T. (1964)., Microanalysis in medical biochemistry Ed. 4J & A, Churchill, London.

Kozhev, A.,; Penelski, I and Panova, V. (1970). Bulgarian sour milk production employing fermentation in bulk. Izv. nauchnoizsted Inst. mlech. Prom. Vidin. **4**, 127-136.

Kumar, M. (2002). Technology and nutritional aspects of yoghurt. Ph.D. Thesis, Banaras Hindu University, Varanasi, India.

Kaminarides, s., Stamou, P. and Massouras, T. (2007). Comparision of the characteristics of set type yoghurt made from ovine milk of different fat content. International J. of Food Sci. and Technol. **42**(9) : 1019-1028.

Lalas, M. and Mantes, A. (1985). Microbiological quality of yoghurt. Deltio Ethnikes Epitropes Galaktos Ellados. **2**(1), 28-29.

Lee, H.; Friend, B.A. and Shahani, K.M. (1988). Factors Affecting the Protein Quality of Yoghurt and Acidophilus Milk. J. Dairy Sci., **71**,323-3213.

MC Millan, H.K. (1990). Thermodynamics. Kinko's Publishing. University of South Califormia, Columbia.

Madan Lal Meena, S.; Gandhi, D.N. and Number Pad, V.K.N.(1978). Studies on selection of starter culture for the manufacture of yoghurt. J. Food Sci. and Technol. **15**(1), 20-21.

Magdesi, T. (1979). Effect of coagulation temperature and addition of dried milk on the quality of yoghurt. Nauchni Trudove, Vissh Institute P.O. Khranitelna; ivkusover Promishlenost. **26**(2), 163-170.

Manjunath, N. and Abraham, M.J. (1986). Yoghurt from goat milk. Asian J. Dairy Res. 5(2), 103-107.

Mann, G.V. (1978). A factor in yoghurt which lowers cholesterol in man. Atherosclerosis **26**,335-340.

Marks, J. and Howard, A.N. (1997). Hypocholesterolacmic effect of milk. Lancet **2**(8041), 763.

Martens, R. (1972). Effect of some variables on consistency and flavour of stirred yoghurt. Revue Agric., Brux. **25**(3), 461-480.

Massey, L.K. (1981). Effect of milk and yoghurt consumption on young adult humen serum lipoprotein. Federation Proceeding **40**(311), 927.

Massey, L.K. and Davidson, M.E. (1983). Effect of lactose content of non fat milk diets on male rat serum lipids and lipoproteins. Annals of Nutrition and Metabolism. **27**(5), 447-454.

Mc Donough, F.E.; Hitchins, A.D. and Wong, N.P. (1982). Effects of yoghurt and freeze dried yoghurt on growth stimulation of rats. J. Food Sci., **47**(5), 1463-1465.

Mc. Namara, D.J.; Lowell, A.E. and Sabb, J.E. (1989). Effect of yoghurt intake on plasma lipid and lipoprotein levels in normolipidemic males. Atherosclerosis, **79** (2-3), 167-171.

Mc Glinchey, N. (1996). Interaction of gelatin, modified starch and milk SNF in heat stabilized yoghurt. Termoestabilizado Alimentacion Equiposy Technologia,. **15**, 123-126(ES).

Mehanna, A.S. and Hefnawy, S.A. (1990). A study to fallow the chemical changes during processing and storage of zobady. Egyptian J. Dairy Sci. **18**(2), 425-434.

Moon, N.J. and Reinbold , G.W. (1978). Compelition in milk cultures of L. bulgaricus and S.thermophilus. J. Milk Food Technol. **39**(2), 337-339.

Moussa, S.Z.; Salama, F.M.M. and Taha, N.A. (1995). Effect of fresh cow's milk and some fermented milk products on rat serum cholesterol, triglycerides, total lipids and lipoprotein levels. Egyptian J. Dairy Sci. **23**(1), 69-80.

Muir, D.D.; Hunter, E.A.; Guillaume, C.; Rychembusch, V. and West, I.G. (1993). Application of response surface methodology to manipulation of the organoleptic properties of set yoghurt. Milchwissenchaft. 48(11), 699-619.

Muir, D.D.; Horne, D.S. and West, I.G. (1997). Genetic polymorphism of bovine k-casein. Effect on textural properties and acceptability of plain set yoghurt. International Dairy Federation. 182-184 ISBN 92-9098026-9.

Navder, K.P.; Fryer, E. and Fryer, H.C. (1990). Effects of skim milk, skim milk yoghurt, orotic acid and uric acid on lipid metabolism in rats. J. Nutritional Biochemistry. 1(12), 640-646.

Nelson, Jonh A. and Trout, G. Malcolm (1964). Judging of Dairy Products, 4th Eds.

Nila, D.V.; Rathi, S.D. and Ingle, V.M. (1987). Studies on the qualities of fruit yoghurt, Indian Food Packer, 41(7), 19-22.

Noeman, A.A. and Shalaby, S.O. (1992). A comparative study between Zabady and acidophilus milk. Egyptian J. Food Sci. 29(Supplement), 43-51.

Nelson, Jahn A. and Trout, G. Malcolm(1964). Judging of dairy products, 4ᵗʰ Edn.

Park, Y.W. (1994) Nutrient and mineral composition of commercial U.S. goat's milk yoghurt. Small Ruminant Res. 13(1), 63-70.

Payers, W.; Rethoms, F.J.M. and Ward, H.D. (1977). The influence of consumption of large quantity of yoghurt or milk on the serum cholesterol concentration. Dairy Sci. Abstr 39(3), 1516p. 174.

Pazakova, J.; Burdova, O.; Turck, P. and Lacikova, A. (1999). Sensorial evaluation of yoghurt produced from cow, ewe and goat milk. Czech J. Food Sci. 17 (1), 31-34.

Poppel, G. and Van-Schaafsma, G. (1996). Cholesterol lowering by a functional yoghurt. In Food Ingredients. Europe Conference Proceedings, 12-14.

Rooney, M.L. (1993). Novel Food packaging. In "Technology of reduced additive foods." ed. J. Smith. Blackie Academics and Professional, 95-120pp.

Rasic, J.L. and Kurman, J. A. (1978). In yoghurt scientific grounds, technology, manufacture and preparation. A Technical Dairy Publishing House, Copenhagen, Denmark.

Rasic, J.L. and Kurman, J.A. (1982). Dairy ingredients in strained bady foods. *XXI Int. Dairy Cong.* (E), **136**.

Rathi, S.D.; Deshmukh, D.K.; Ingle, U.M. and Syed, H.M. (1990). Studies on the physico-chemical properties of freeze dried dahi. Indian J. Dairy Sci. 43(2), 249-251.

Real Del Sol, E.; Rocamora, Y.; Ortega, O. Cabrena, M.C.; Casals, C.; Chang, L. and Espinosa, B. (2000). Yoghurt (manufactured) from buffalo and cow milk. Alimentaria. 37(310), 45-48.

Resubal, L.E.; Coallado, E.R.; Emata, O.C. and Lapiz, E.S. (1987). Quality of yoghurt made from fresh skim milk and fortified with skim milk powder. *Philipipine Agriculturist.* 70(3-4), 171-177.

Richter, R.L. ; Watts, C.W.; Gehrig, T.C.; Cheshier, K. and Dill, C.W. (1979). The relationship of milk fat, milk solids-not-fat and sugar to consumer acceptance of plain yoghurt. *J. Dairy, Sci.* **62**(Suppl., I), 205-206.

Robinson, R.K. (1977). A dairy product for the future concentrated yoghurt. *South African J. Dairy Technol.* **9**(2), 59-61.

Robinson, R.K. and Tamime, A.Y. (1986). The role of protein in yoghurt. *Developments in food proteins.* **4**, 1-35.

Robinson, R.K. (1987). Survival of Lactobacillus acidophilus in fermented products. Suid-Afrikanse Tydskrif Vir Suiwelkunde. **19**(1), 25-27.

Robinson, R.K. (1988). Cultures for yoghurt their selection and use. Dairy Industries International. **59**(7), 15-19.

Roos, N.M.; Schouten, G.; Katan, M.B. and de-Ross, N.M. (1999). Yoghurt enriched with Lactobacillus acidophillus does not lower blood lipids in healthy men and women with normal to borderline high serum cholesterol levels. European J. Clin. Nutr. **53**(4), 277-280.

Rossouw, J.E.; Burger, E.; Van der Vyver, P. and Ferreira, J.J. (1981). The effect of skim milk, yoghurt and full cream on human serum lipids. *Am. J. Clin. Nutr.* **34**, 315-356.

Ruddel, L.L. and Moris, M.D. (1973). Determination of cholesterol using O-phthalaldehyde *J. Lipids Res.* **14**, 364.

Rhanna, R. (2001). The emerging internal dairy marketing scenario and the chalanges of quality cited in sustainable animal production. Edited by singh R.A.,Singh, R.P. and Khanna, A.S, (2001). SSARM, CCS, HAU, Hissar, pp. 197-207.

Rossi, E.A.; Cavallini, D.C.V.; Carlos, 1.Z; Vendramini, R.C.;*Damaso*, A.R. and Front de Valdez, g. (2008). Intake of isoflavon-supplemented soy yoghurt permented with Enterococcus faecium lowers serum total cholesterol and non-HDL cholesterol of hypercholesterolemic rats. European Food Res. and Technol. **228**(2) : 275-282.

Salem, S.A.; Attia, J.A.; Godda, E. and Kumar, M.S. (1994). Studies on frozen yoghurt. Effect of using high level of fat with different inocula of starter. Egyptian *J. Food Sci.* **22**(1), 27-39.

Sanyal, M.K. and Yadav, P.L. (1986). Sensory evaluation of dahi made from the milk of cross-bred calves. *Indiay Dairyman.* **38**(9), 465.

Saxena, E. (2000). Dynamics of demand for milk in this millenium. *Indian Dairyman.* **2**II(12), 47.

Shakeel, A. and Thompkinson, D.K. (1994). Influence of composition and processing parameters on curd tension of fruit flavoured filled yoghurt. *Indian J. Dairy Sci.* **47**(8) : 695-697.

Shaker, R.R. ; Jumah, R.Y. and Abu-Jdyik, B. (2000). Rheological properties of plain yoghurt during coagulation process : Impact of fat content and pre heat treatment of milk. *J. Food Engg.* **44**(3), 175-180.

Tosikowsky, F. (1996). cheese and fermented milk foods, Edward brothers Inc, Ann. Arbor, 128.

Vedamuthu, E. R. (1991). The yoghurt story-past present and future. Dairy Food Environ. Sanit. 11:202-514.

Yuji Nakazawa and Akiyoshi Hosono (1992). Functions of fermented milk-challanges for the health sciences. I. Edition, Elsevier applied science, London.

Yeganehzad, S.; Mazaheri-Tehrani, M. and Shahidi, F. (2007). Studying microbial, physico-chemical and sensory properties of directly concentrated probiotic yoghurt. African J. of Agri. Res. **2**(8) : 366-369.